Clean Food Diet

The 21-Day Clean Eating Guide
to Lose Weight,
Reduce Inflammation,
Boost Energy and
Look Better Naked

Melodee Meyer

Published by
Master Mel Productions
122 E. Gutierrez Street
Santa Barbara, CA 93101

Manufactured in the United States of America, or in the United Kingdom when distributed elsewhere.

Cover design by: Melodee Meyer/Vittoria Cutbirth/Julia McPherson
Photo of Melodee Meyer by: Stephanie Westover

Ebook: 978-0-9986496-0-3
Ingram Spark Softcover: 978-0-9986496-1-0
Createspace: ISBN-13:978-1548662493
Createspace: ISBN-10:1548662496

A portion of the proceeds of this book will go to support Heal the Ocean, a non-profit organization committed to ending ocean pollution.

Author's URL: http://www.MasterMel.com

Disclaimer

The Clean Food Diet is not intended as medical advice. The reader is advised to consult a physician regarding his or her health, especially for symptoms that may require diagnosis or medical attention.

Acknowledgements

It takes a village to raise a child . . . and to write a book. This one is no exception.

"I am forever grateful to the many teachers in my life who fed me, taught me, and inspired me, in (and out) of the kitchen."

Thanks to my mom who made cooking look easy by whipping up magical meals and delicious Dutch treats for a family of six from seemingly nothing. Thank you, Dad, for showing me how to raise a cow, and then how to barbeque it properly.

It was Chef Anita Krissel, professional culinary consultant and foodie extraordinaire, who generously taught me how to make food the star of the meal by allowing the natural flavors to shine through. Thanks to her, my friends and family think I'm a genius in the kitchen, when all I do is use the best-quality products I can get my hands on, and then season them with freshly ground salt and pepper. True story.

I also want to thank Chef Isa Bourbon for her Zen attitude and amazing recipes, which bring joy and life to all she does. Her delicious food fills the belly and warms the heart.

I am grateful to my husband, Dave Wheaton, who loves to be in the kitchen and kept me from starving... as I wrote about food.

Thanks to my editor, Hilary Klein, who not only tested my grammar but some of the recipes as well. Torrie Cutbirth is a saint for putting up with me and pulling everything together for this manuscript on a crazy deadline. And thanks to the rest of my team, Amanda Arcuri, Rachael Bourke, Christian Sierra, and Austin Curtis, for all your love and support.

And last but not least, I want to thank all of the KUT students over the years who took the challenge to transform their bodies and their lives by exercising and following a Clean Food Diet. I am so proud of you and humbled to hear your success stories and be a part of your journey to greater health and abundance. You make it all worthwhile!

Contents

Foreword

By Dr. Anne Marie Fine

As I was growing up, I nearly died several times from severe asthma and spent a lot of time in the emergency rooms of hospitals. In my twenties, the discovery by an integrative doctor of my extensive food allergies transformed my life by pinpointing the many foods that were making me chronically ill.

Chronic disease, by definition, is an incurable disease with significant negative impact on the quality of life. It's also on the rise. According to the Centers for Disease Control, 78% of Americans over the age of 55 have 1 chronic disease, 47% have 2 or more, and 19% suffer from 3 or more. Furthermore, autoimmune diseases now affect nearly 50 million Americans, predominantly women. And more than two-thirds of Americans are overweight or obese.

How did we get to this point?

My own experience with chronic disease has shown me that the biggest culprits that have led us into poor health and obesity are the processed foods that comprise most of our diets.

At first I was quite depressed to think that I had to eliminate my allergenic foods — all the good tasting ones like wheat, eggs, and dairy. I thought I would be living on rice crackers for the rest of my life. It didn't occur to me that there was a tasty world of fresh, non-processed food out there. But when I began to eat a lot of vegetables, fruits, non-gluten grains, and fish, my health improved.

I was able to get off all prescription drugs, and my energy skyrocketed. Best of all, my asthma vanished!

Melodee Meyer overcame her own obstacles to healing by switching to a diet that includes only "clean" foods, a diet that focuses exclusively on whole and natural foods and steers clear of processed foods. Her approach to eating, masterful in its simplicity, has proven to be a key strategy in preventing and reversing chronic and autoimmune diseases, losing weight, and gaining energy.

We now know that many of today's medical problems can be reversed with lifestyle changes. As an integrative doctor I recommend the Clean Food Diet to my patients as a part of a health restoration that begins in the gut. Because most of our immune system resides in the gut, a poor diet wreaks havoc on it, resulting in many of the chronic diseases and health problems of today.

Furthermore, the constant hunger and cravings we are seeing stem from the fact that our bodies are literally crying out for nutrients as we fill up on processed foods full of sugar, artificial flavorings, and additives — ingredients our bodies neither recognize nor need, and which cannot sustain good health.

Melodee's clear, concise, accessible book provides guidance on what constitutes a clean diet, why it will work, and how to assemble fresh ingredients into tasty, doable menus and meal plans. The Clean Food Diet provides an abundance of nutrients and fiber in a form that the human body recognizes and can use, the way we ate before fast food franchises and factory food.

Instead of an exclusionary diet prohibiting entire food groups and resulting in feelings of deprivation and sacrifice, the Clean Food Diet focuses on delicious, generous, satisfying meals of quality wholesome fruits and vegetables, along with healthy fats and meats that are organic, free range, and free from the antibiotics and medicines often given to commercially-raised, confined animals. You will also be getting all the vitamins, minerals, micronutrients, and phytochemicals that food contains before processing destroys them.

The Clean Food Diet will educate and inform you on how to overcome your own health challenges and become your best self. Don't settle for anything less. Excess weight, stomach aches, poor digestion, joint pain, fatigue, and illness are not your birthright. Abundant energy and robust health will facilitate your ability to live your dreams. I highly recommend that you follow this guide and its 21-day plan to lose weight, gain energy, reduce inflammation — and look great naked.

Congratulations Melodee on your brilliant and elegant contribution to Clean Eating!

Dr. Anne Marie Fine

In addition to her private practice, Dr. Fine is a highly respected researcher, bestselling author, and sought-after international speaker. With a lifelong commitment to unlocking the secrets and science of aging beautifully, she is also the Founder and CEO of Fine Natural Products, dedicated to formulating non-toxic anti-aging beauty products.

www.DrAnneMarieFine.com

Introduction

It is health that is real wealth and not pieces of gold and silver.
-Mahatma Gandhi

This is a short book. Eating clean food is simple, so let's keep it that way. I assume that you are reading this book because you want to look better and feel better, and you don't have a lot of time to waste talking about it.

If you like to get to the point, cut to the chase, and drop to the bottom line, then this is the book for you. However, you can't just read about it — you've got to do it! Results come from consistently taking action and this is your opportunity to upgrade your health . . . regardless of where you are starting from.

In service of moving quickly, this is a "What" book, and not so much of a "Why" book. We are going to go over WHAT the Clean Food Diet is, rather than go into a lot of the reasons WHY this is the best way to eat your way healthy. I am going to shortcut this whole process for you by providing the plan that I have used to help thousands of people lose weight, reduce inflammation, boost energy, and look better naked (or so they tell me).

"Why it Works" would be a long book and, remember, this is a short book. I like science and data as much as the next person, so please visit my website (MasterMel.com) to find some of my favorite resources for you to pour through.

I also encourage you to do as much research as you need to feel confident in your new eating plan.

The most important question for you to be successful on this journey is your Big Why: Why are you here? Why do you want to be healthy? Why is this important to you? Your Big Why will help you get through the challenges that are ahead for all of us who choose a new destiny for ourselves.

So spend the time. Ask the big questions. Figure it out. Knowing your Big Why is work you will have to do on your own because after all, this is a short book.

My Big Why

He who has a why to live for can bear almost any how.
- Friedrich Nietzsche

I thought it was normal to need to lie down after eating. Every time I ate, I would have such a pain in my gut, along with gas and bloating. And yet I just accepted that's how it was.

As a teenager, I had a lot of shame around food and my weight. Bulimia was my dirty little secret, and I thought that this pain was somehow related to that. The one time I brought up the pain to my doctor, he told me it was a stress-related ulcer and sent me home with an antibiotic prescription, which made it worse.

Thankfully, I was able to get the help I needed for my eating disorder, but I could not lose weight or that nagging pain. I would have to go lie on the couch after eating, or if I was out, I would go lie down in the ladies room. Yes, on the floor of a public bathroom — that's how bad it was. But it was the only thing that would help the pain subside.

I figured it had something to do with my digestion, but no one seemed to know what to do about it. I would get advice like, "Eat more fiber," which I did. I ate oatmeal every morning, I ate beans and brown rice, and I took several fiber supplements.

There was a time when I was doing a psyllium drink three times a day and got so big and bloated that I looked six months pregnant. I didn't feel better, I felt worse.

Perhaps it was what I was eating? So I became a vegetarian. Then a vegan. I even tried eating a raw food diet, thinking I just needed to try harder and be more extreme. And yet I continued to experience gut-wrenching pain.

Sometimes the pain would manifest as constipation, and other times it turned into spontaneous diarrhea. Nice, right? I remember one time walking down the main street of a small town that shall remain nameless (just in case someone was there), feeling the rumble and panicking to find a bathroom. I did not get to one in time . . . I don't need to go into a lot of detail on this, but let's just say it was scary and very humiliating.

Oh, and did I mention the gas? I thought everyone had gas so smelly it could make a grown man's eyes water and a small dog's nose bleed. Then one day I was standing in line at the drugstore, and I discreetly passed a little "normal" gas, and a child turned to his mom and said, "Ewwww, Mommy, did something die?"

The doctor tested me for food allergies, but the results came back negative. "According to the tests, you are perfectly healthy," I was told. Great, thanks. I had self-diagnosed myself as being lactose intolerant because of my volatile reaction to all things dairy, but my doctor argued with me. "You should be fine eating anything you like," he said.

Other doctors diagnosed me with Irritable Bowel Syndrome (IBS), diverticulitis, ulcers, volvulus (intestinal obstruction), low thyroid, and hormone deficiencies, to name a few. They gave me prescriptions but didn't have a good explanation as to why. When the medications didn't work, I resigned myself to the idea that this was my normal: overweight, chronic abdominal pain, constipation with bouts of diarrhea, severe bloating, fatigue, and terrible gas. I craved sweets all the time and blamed myself for not being impeccable on my diet. Secretly, I felt the pain was somehow my punishment for not being perfect.

The silver lining in all of this was that my own health problems fueled my desire to learn more. I dove into a career in health and fitness, studied psychology, nutrition, and martial arts, always looking for new solutions. The message became clear: Stop poisoning yourself with toxic foods and start feeding yourself what your body actually needs.

So that's what I did. I started eating cleaner, simpler, and closer to the farm. I ate more of what could be found in nature and cut out what was made in a factory. I changed the way I ate and instantly felt better. Instantly. I lost weight. I lost the gas, the bloating, and the doubling over in pain. I stopped getting tired in the middle of the day and stopped my ongoing struggle with food.

I went from feeling betrayed by my body and hating what I saw in the mirror every day to loving my body and enjoying my healthy life.

Teaching what I learned to my fitness and martial arts students became my passion, and the results were incredible! People lost weight, reversed autoimmune diseases, stopped the incessant cravings, and absolutely transformed their lives.

Self Mastery

I have worked in the personal development field for many years and have experienced more people having personal breakthroughs by changing their food than anything else. My Big Why for sharing this information with you is to help you on your own journey of self-mastery. Learning about your body and how your mind functions best is key. In the Self Mastery System that I teach, proper nutrition through clean eating is foundational. Nothing else matters if you don't have your health; it is the platform that all other personal and professional development builds on.

Now don't get me wrong. Although taking care of our body is a priority, we are not our bodies. We are not our minds. We are spiritual beings who have a body and a mind. That being said, it becomes our responsibility to care for our body and our mind in such a way that we can live a life to our greatest potential and for our highest purpose.

The Clean Food Diet became my ticket to amazing health, and it is what I have used with thousands of people to help them create the life they want, in a body they love. Don't take my word for it. Do it for 21 days and see for yourself.

You deserve it.

For more information about self-mastery and how you can have the life you want, in a body you love, doing work that matters, please visit my website (www.MasterMel.com). I would love to hear your story and support you in any way I can.

With much love,

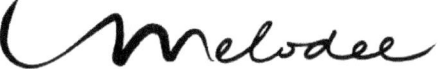

This book includes free training, more recipes, downloadable food lists and community support so you can fast-track your health and love that body of yours NOW! Get it all for free at: www.MasterMel.com/CFD

I want to hear from you! Connect with me here:

@MelodeeMeyer

3 Good Reasons to Eat Clean

You can't wait for inspiration. You have to go after it with a club.
- Jack London

Although I said we would not be going into "Why It Works" (too much), I do want to go over three important reasons why you will want to do the Clean Food Diet: healthy digestion, balanced hormones, and stabilized blood sugar. Doesn't sound sexy? Well, it is the failure of these three pillars of health that is wreaking havoc in your body, perhaps without you even knowing it, so read on. Or not. You can always jump to the Clean Food Diet Lists and just get started. However, this information will help support your Big Why.

1. A Healthy Gut

I cannot overstate how important the gut is to health. In fact, I would go so far as to say that an unhealthy gut is the root of dis-ease. We come in contact with viruses and bacteria every day, which could potentially harm us, but our bodies are designed in such a way to deal with these dangers through proper digestion and elimination. Also, a healthy digestive system is necessary for us to absorb the nutrients from our food.

Unfortunately, there are stats out there that reveal nearly 80% of the current population has a dangerous condition called leaky gut. It is almost impossible to diagnose, because we are busy treating the symptoms, not the cause.

So what is leaky gut?

The gut, which is the gastrointestinal tract, is like a complex food processor. It breaks down food that is either absorbed or eliminated from the body. Along with processing food, the gut has the vital role of being the selective barrier between us and the outside environment.

The cells in the gut's lining are connected by tight junctions. These junctions are the part of the gut that act as a barrier, deciding what gets through and what gets denied. Basically, the gut lining is like a bouncer that lets in the good stuff like nutrients and water, and keeps out the bad like pathogens, toxins, and antigens. While this process is simple enough, sometimes those tight junctions don't do their job, and things get in that aren't supposed to. When this happens, those bad substances crash the party. They leak into the bloodstream and make a mess of the place, which happens to be our body. This is leaky gut.

Leaky gut is a syndrome also known as intestinal permeability. The gut is like a tube, and like most tubes, it can develop a leak. When the tight junctions of the lining are compromised and allow potentially harmful or antigenic compounds into our body, then all of that gross stuff like undigested food particles, toxins, and bacteria can leak through our intestines and into our bloodstream. When these things make their way into our bodies, it can cause a great deal of problems such as inflammation and ultimately an autoimmune response.

Leaky gut is the first step towards autoimmune disease, which can cause a multitude of complications. Some of these are celiac disease, inflammatory bowel disease, and irritable bowel syndrome, as well as digestive issues such as gas, bloating, and diarrhea. It's also known to cause asthma, food allergies, and food intolerances. If that weren't enough, leaky gut has also been linked to autism, lupus, narcolepsy, depression, Alzheimer's, arthritis, obesity, skin issues like eczema and acne, and psoriasis, infertility, type 1 diabetes, headaches, Crohn's disease, poor immune system, multiple sclerosis, chronic fatigue and even anxiety. Now how is THAT for a list?!

There are many things that can cause leaky gut, including stress, poor sleeping habits, and non-inflammatory drugs. However, in most cases it is caused by what we eat. Certain foods cause inflammation and irritation, which not only lead to leaky gut but ultimately lead to autoimmune disease. Here are some of the main food culprits of leaky gut:

- Gluten (wheat and other grains) can damage your intestinal lining.
- Processed foods and GMOs are high in lectins, which are sugar-binding proteins that attach to the digestive lining, causing inflammation.
- Sugar creates toxins that can eat a hole in your intestinal wall.
- The pasteurization of dairy destroys vital enzymes, making lactose hard to digest.
- Legumes contain anti-nutrients and other substances that increase leakage.
- Too much alcohol reduces zinc, which is a critical pro-gut nutrient, along with causing intestinal inflammation.

When we continue to eat these leaky-gut-inducing foods over and over again, an inflammatory sequence persists, and the gut is unable to heal. Therefore, it's essential to provide the nutrients necessary to help the gut repair itself. This can be done by cleaning up your diet. You just have to cut out the toxic foods and start eating the whole foods you'll find on the Clean Food Diet.

Clean Food Diet foods include fruits, vegetables, pasture-raised meat, seafood, nuts and seeds, and healthy fats. Removing the processed foods that damage your gut and replacing them with these nutrient-dense, healing foods will rejuvenate the lining of the intestinal wall and help your leaky gut get back on track.

Adding probiotics and fermented foods can help, as will moderate exercise, stress management, and plenty of sleep.

Leaky gut is rarely diagnosed, and the symptoms are left to be treated one by one. Or worse, an autoimmune disease ensues and eclipses attention from the original culprit. Eat clean and help your gut get healthy.

2. Balanced Hormones

A huge benefit of the Clean Food Diet is that it helps balance the hormone levels in the body and keeps them running efficiently. But how does that affect us day to day?

Hormones are the body's messengers. Their role is to deliver crucial information from specific glands such as the thyroid, adrenal, and pituitary glands to tissue and organ cells throughout the body. When people hear hormones, they often think of the sex hormones such as estrogen, progesterone, and testosterone; but there are other hormones like melatonin, dopamine, and serotonin. Did you know that leptin, insulin, cortisol, adrenaline, and histamine are all hormones as well? There are many more hormones that our body uses to signal different functions throughout the body.

Hormones help regulate our physical and psychological functions. Some of these functions are digestion, metabolism, respiration, growth (when to start and stop growing), stress (like fight-or-flight response), mood, blood pressure, appetite, and pain.

When our hormones are out of whack, they can really mess with our bodies. Hormone imbalances can cause poor sleep patterns, weaken our immune system, make us really hungry and crave things, and make us tired all the time. When our hormones are out of balance, we gain weight easily, our libido is lower, and we have sweating or digestive problems. If that's not bad enough, hormone imbalances also cause anxiety, depression, belly fat, and a loss of muscle mass.

When our hormones are well balanced, everything works a lot better. Balanced hormones keep us healthy and happy; they aid in weight loss, support our thyroid, boost energy, help recovery from exercise, improve our mood, and so much more. Inspired to keep your hormones balanced yet?

The Clean Food Diet consists of eating foods that help maintain hormonal harmony — specifically foods that are high in Omega-3 fats. Omega-3s have been shown to help reduce inflammation and arthritis, and help maintain a healthy metabolism.

They can be found in coconut milk; avocados; plant oils such as avocado oil, olive oil, coconut oil, and fish oil; and many types of nuts. Just as important as eating the foods that support our hormonal system, is NOT eating the foods that make our hormones run amuck.

Foods known to negatively affect our hormones include:

- Grains and grain products such as barley, buckwheat, corn, millet, oats, rye, rice, quinoa, wheat, breads, and pastas.
- Legumes such as different types of beans, peas, peanuts, and soy (including tofu).
- Dairy such as cheese, milk, and cottage cheese.
- Many starches (i.e. potatoes).
- Sugar, which not only refers to table sugar and candy, but also many types of sweeteners such as honey, syrup, and agave. (Yes, even natural forms of sugar can mess with hormones, but we'll get to that later.)
- Soft drinks, fruit juices, energy drinks, and smoothies, even though we've been told that these things are really good for us.
- Processed foods. (Does it have a label? It's processed.)

By eating the Clean Food Diet, we return to how our bodies were designed to eat. We need good nutrition to repair imbalances so that our hormones can do their job and keep us healthy and happy.

3. Stabilized Blood Sugar

Cholesterol has been villainized as the cause of heart disease. This is not exactly correct. We need cholesterol, so much so, our body actually makes cholesterol. However, when cholesterol combines with calcium, fat, and other substances in the blood to form plaque, and that plaque builds up, there is a problem. It is high blood sugar that helps cause this plaque build-up.

High blood sugar coats our red blood cells and makes them stiff and sticky. These cells interfere with circulation and cause cholesterol to pile up. It's not cholesterol that is the problem, it's those sticky cells that block the way. It takes years for this damage to appear, and it starts to affect fragile blood vessels first, like the eyes, feet, and kidneys.

Too much sugar in our system turns into obesity, hyperactivity, tooth decay, metabolic syndrome, cardiovascular disease, addiction, and diabetes. In other words, it shortens our lives and diminishes our health. The problem is that in today's world, sugar is everywhere.

Sugar is a type of carbohydrate that can be found in fruits, veggies, starches, grains, and dairy. (Sugar cannot be found in proteins or fat.) It can also be found in almost every kind of processed food. Read your labels to see for yourself. There are many names for sugar. If a word ends in "ide" or "ose," it's sugar: sucrose, fructose, maltose, dextrose, monosaccharide, etc. HFCS stands for high fructose corn syrup. Also, ingredients using fancy words like syrup, juice, nectar, glaze, and crystals are code for sugar.

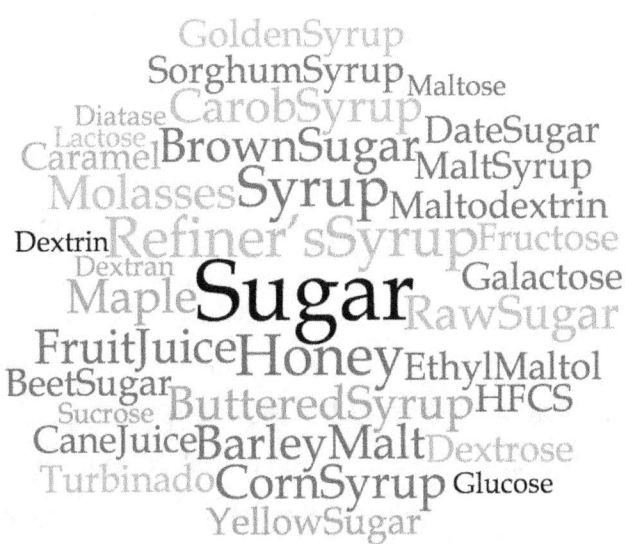

On labels, ingredients are listed in order of quantity, so manufacturers sometimes use many different kinds of sugars so that sugar isn't the first ingredient listed. However, when you add them all together, there is more sugar in the product than anything else.

Have you looked at your labels yet? Yep, there's sugar in your marinara sauce, your peanut butter, and your ketchup. Sugar loves to hide in salad dressing, diet snacks, soups, instant oatmeal, chips, cereals, and yogurt. If it's got a label, it probably has some kind of sugar. Frankly, sugar makes food taste better and therefore sell better.

What a lot of people don't realize is that sugar as a commodity hasn't been around for very long. It's only been available to common people since the 18th century. The intake of sugar in our diet has progressively increased over the last 100 years, coincidently, at a similar rate to the rise of obesity, sickness, and disease.

Sugar isn't all bad. When we have it every once in a while, our body knows exactly how to deal with it and can actually use it for our benefit. Sugar is a carbohydrate and carbs are very useful. Our body uses carbs to make glucose, which is the body's major source for fuel. The body can use the glucose immediately or can store it in the liver or the muscles. However, what's interesting is that the body doesn't actually need dietary carbs from food for glucose. It can convert protein to glucose — although the process takes a little bit longer.

Carbohydrates are comprised of three different nutrients: sugar, starches, and dietary fiber. Simple carbs, such as those found in sweets, milk, and even fruit, convert quickly to glucose, much faster than complex carbs like those from veggies. What that means for you is, every time you consume simple carbs, the glucose gets into your bloodstream quickly and can spike your blood sugar levels.

Another issue with simple carbs is that they displace the nutrition that comes from real food. Every time you eat simple carbs like breads and pastas, you're not eating veggies and proteins, which have a much greater level of nutrition. So here we are. Carbs are important, yet we don't need to get them from sugar. But wait a second, don't we need to eat carbs for energy? Don't you need one of those energy drinks or energy bars in order to keep your energy up? Well, it depends on what kind of energy you want.

There are two different sources of energy in the body: sugar and fat.

If I were going to light a dark room with a match, it would light up for a second, and then the light would go out. That's not sustainable energy — it's up and then it's down, very much like your energy level is on sugar. If I light a candle instead, the room is lit and will stay that way for the life of the candle, very much like the kind of energy that comes when burning fat. Fat is a much more consistent and sustainable choice for energy than sugar.

Stored body fat is an excellent source of useable energy. The problem is, you can't burn sugar and fat at the same time. You're either burning sugar or fat. It's like having a car that's either gas or its diesel. It's burning one or the other — you can't burn both of them at the same time. If you have excess sugar in your blood, you can't burn stored body fat. So if you want to lose the fat, you must stop eating the sugar and level out those blood sugar levels so your body can start converting your stored body fat into energy.

Becoming a fat burner can be very challenging, and you have to be patient with yourself. But I want you to know that it's totally worth it. If you eliminate sugar, and your body starts going to that stored body fat for energy, then you will be amazed at what happens. Your cravings will start to go away, you'll feel more grounded, and you'll start to have more energy. You just won't believe how great it feels. But, like I said, to get to that point can be a little challenging, and you might have to white-knuckle it for a bit. I've seen it happen in as little as two days, but I've also seen it take two and even as long as three weeks.

You will need self-control to keep away from the sugar for a period of time, but eventually it gets easier. Hang in there, you can do it!

Just imagine: by eliminating excess sugar, you will reduce cravings, avoid mood and energy swings, reduce the risk of disease, and become a fat-burning machine!

Another Diet, Really?

The first thing you lose on a diet is brain mass.
-Margaret Cho

For years I have preached, "Stop Dieting!" at the top of my lungs, so imagine the mumbling I heard when I announced I was releasing this Clean Food Diet book. Had I changed my mind about diets? Of course not.

Diet in the typical sense is the restriction of food in order to lose weight. There's a reason DIET has the word DIE in it. It's not a good idea. Diet is the last resort of torture you agree to endure in order to fit into a dress that you don't like and will never wear again, so you can go to an event that you really don't care about, with self-absorbed, entitled people who drive you crazy. Or maybe that's just me.

Diets don't work. Studies show that 95% of diets fail, and most people regain their weight plus more in one to five years. In fact, in a study UCLA did, they found that two years following a diet, 83% of the dieters had gained back more weight than they had lost. Yikes. Traci Mann, UCLA associate professor of psychology and lead author of the study concluded, "Diets do not lead to sustained weight loss or health benefits for the majority of people." I'd say.

You've oooh'd and aaah'd over all the before-and-after photos you've seen, where fat girl becomes skinny girl and wondered how you could do that too, right? What you want to see is the after-after photo.

That's the tell-tale. Anyone can lose weight but how does one keep it off?

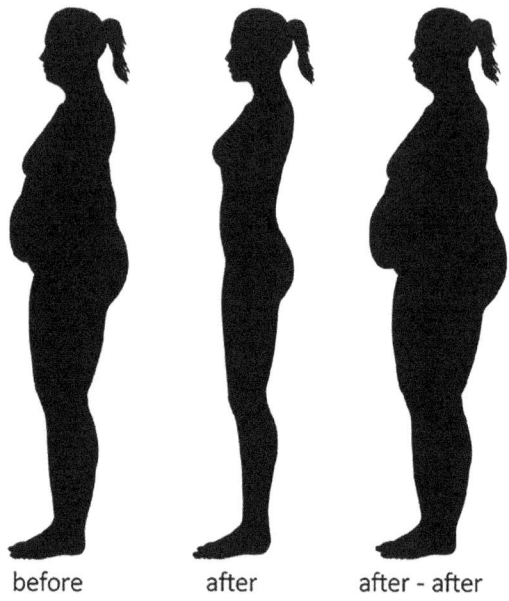

before   after   after - after

The definition of diet we are using for this book is "habitual nourishment." What foods do you habitually nourish your body with? You have the opportunity to examine, and even change, how you nourish your body with the Clean Food Diet.

If you treat this guide like another one of your adventures of deprivation, you will have the same disastrous results as you got from those other diets. Stop it! Yo-yo dieting is one of the worst things you can do for your health and your waistline.

If however, you are looking for a way to get healthy, shed excess body fat, and keep it off effortlessly, then this Clean Food Diet guide is for you. Want to maintain your health or reverse some negative health challenges you are experiencing? This is for you as well! The key is in the definition of diet as *habitual nourishment.*

To enjoy the long-term benefits of sustained health, eating clean food has to become a habit and a lifestyle.

And once you have developed the habit of nourishing your body with clean food, your after-after photo will only get better.

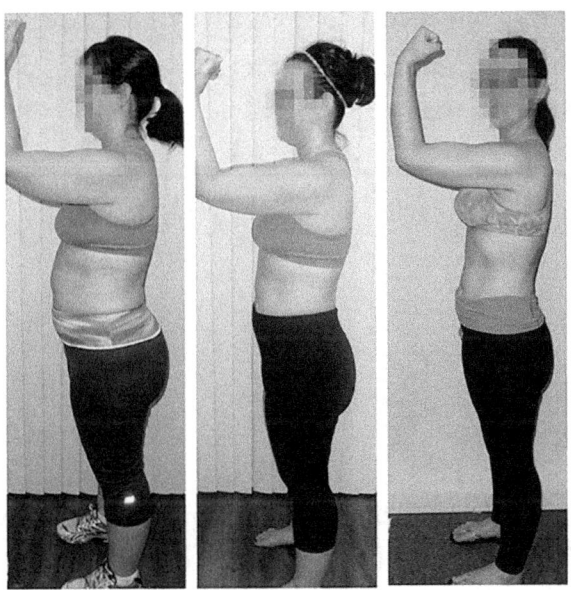

The Pareto Principle

Vilfredo Pareto was an Italian economist who observed that 80% of Italy's income was received by 20% of the Italian population. An engineer and quality management thought leader, Joseph M. Juran coined the principle, when he also saw that most of the results in any situation are determined by a small number of causes.

How does this principle affect you? Probably in more ways than you can imagine, but for the purposes of this book, I propose the following in regards to your health: The 20% of your day that is spent preparing, cooking, and eating food will result in 80% of your results. It is that important.

If you want to lose weight, you've got to change what you eat. If you want to reverse disease and promote healing, you've got to change the quality of your food. If you want to have more energy, you've got to change your fuel.

That is why we are going to focus on FOOD in this book. However, I want to take a few minutes to acknowledge what accounts for the other 80% that is also important to your health.

There are several nutrients that your body needs besides food:

WATER

Water regulates our body temperature, transports nutrients, flushes out toxins, lubricates joints, hydrates and strengthens muscles, makes skin clearer and brighter, improves cognitive function, and acts as a shock absorber for the brain and spinal cord. Oh, and it curbs appetite.

We are made up of 60% water, and it is an essential nutrient to every cell of our bodies. In fact, our hearts and our brains are composed of 73% water — so imagine what happens when we don't drink enough of the stuff.

To make sure you are getting enough water, a good rule of thumb is to drink half of your body weight in fluid ounces. For example, if you weigh 160 pounds, you will drink 80 fluid ounces of water per day.

SLEEP

Sleep is probably the most underrated health factor by the most people. Quality sleep is important for every aspect of our lives, physically, mentally, and emotionally.

We need sleep to balance hormones, regulate blood sugar; strengthen immunity; and repair cells, organs, tissues, and blood vessels. Without good sleep, we can't grow properly, our brains can't work effectively, and weight loss is nearly impossible.

Good quality sleep hygiene is important to cultivate. Most people need about eight hours of sleep, so let's get to bed!

EXERCISE

Our bodies were designed to move, not sit around all day. When we move, we actually dictate how our genes are expressed. There are the obvious benefits, such as strengthening muscles and building bone and cardiovascular health, yet exercise affects the body in many other ways as well.

For one thing, exercise optimizes insulin receptor sensitivity, which prevents chronic disease and is important for overall health. Exercise also improves circulation, metabolism, sexual function, emotional wellbeing, clearer skin, greater lung capacity, and that's just the beginning. Don't even get me started on what exercise does for the brain.

Everything in your life will improve with exercise. Regular exercise was found to increase productivity and happiness on any given day, according to a 2012 study published in Neuroscience Journal. The study found that a little exercise each day was better than a lot of exercise only once or twice per week.

Find something fun and active to do. Make sure you get a minimum of 30 minutes of exercise doing something you enjoy. Every day.

MINDFULNESS

The ability to focus your awareness on the present moment, while accepting your thoughts, feelings, and physical sensations, is called mindfulness and it is a skill that you can develop with practice.

Mindfulness is one of the most important skills you can learn that will balance your mood, clear your thoughts, improve your relationships, lower stress, and reduce the risk of illness.

There are several ways to cultivate mindfulness and one of the most effective is meditation. There are a lot of verifiable studies that demonstrate the benefits of meditation for pain management, increased creativity and brain function, better self-esteem, improved memory, greater productivity, and reversal of the aging process. Om….

Take a journey inside — spend a minimum of ten minutes a day to breathe, meditate, walk in nature, journal, or some other enjoyable (non)activity.

FUN

Many health problems are caused by stress, including depression, anxiety, heart disease, sleep issues, weight gain, and poor digestion. The good news is, laughter and fun are proven to be an effective way of coping with stress.

Yes, fun could be called Stress Management but that doesn't sound like much, uh, fun. It is so incredibly important to our health to laugh, love, be positive, and experience joy that it qualifies for its own book.

Even a simple smile releases endorphins, which are neurotransmitter hormones that send a message of satisfaction and confidence to the brain. Laughter releases serotonin, a hormone that produces an all-natural high. Sound good? It is.

Smiling, laughing, and having fun generate a sense of optimism, which will help you live more than seven years longer, according to a recent study. Dr. Becca Levy, a psychologist at Yale University states, "Having an optimistic attitude towards aging is better than having low blood pressure and cholesterol levels."

Funny thing is, you don't even have to feel like smiling or laughing to benefit. Even forcing a smile or faking a laugh will positively affect your emotions. Hahahahahaha! How fun.

Remember, all of these physical, emotional, spiritual, and mental nutrients are super important, and yet they account for only 20% of your results. But now, let's turn our focus to what will provide you with the other 80% — eating clean food.

What Is Clean Food?

If man made it, don't eat it.
- Jack LaLanne

Eating "clean" is a way that magazine editors, wellness professionals, and celebrities have tried to describe a popular movement in healthy eating without branding it. Maybe all the cool names like the Zone or South Beach were taken. Regardless, there seems to be many different ideas as to what clean eating actually entails.

For the purposes of this book, we will define it as such:

Clean Food is real food that can be eaten in its natural state.

Eating a Clean Food Diet like our ancestors did for thousands of years is sometimes referred to by several other names. Some people call it Paleo, which stands for Paleolithic, referring to the period in our history when we were hunters and gatherers. Some call it low carb, Atkins, Weston A. Price, or gluten/grain/dairy free. Although the Clean Food Diet has similarities to all of these things, I like the simplicity of "eating clean" and find that name brings up less opposition.

For instance, the Paleo Diet has come under scrutiny, because we can't possible mimic the foods that cavemen (and cavewomen) ate. The fruit and veggies we enjoy today are a far cry from those original plants, to be sure, thanks to modern agriculture tinkering. Does that mean we throw the baby out with the bath water? Of course not. The same goes for the diets outlined by cardiologist Robert Atkins and dentist Weston A. Price. They helped us learn a lot by examining the diets of people who did not suffer from the health problems and obesity we see today.

That being said, I think it is important to keep it simple and not get into too much dogma. Clean food is real food that can be eaten in its natural state. It's not a religion; it's a guide to reclaiming our bodies and our health.

Real Food vs Pretend Food

Real food can be found in nature and is designed for the body to digest. It can be hunted or foraged, and it is how mankind has been eating since the beginning of time. In our modern society, hunting and gathering is done at the supermarket, so it becomes trickier to know if the food we find there is actually real.

Pretend food is made by man or machine and is designed for profit. It is highly processed and cannot be eaten in its natural state. The three big clues that quickly identify pretend foods are: they usually come in a box or package, they don't rot quickly, and they need a label to identify what is in them.

Let's be clear. Just because you can put something in your mouth, chew it up, and have it work its way through your body, doesn't mean that it is food. Agreed? If I eat my phone bill, that doesn't make it food. Even if someone writes a cute jingle, covers it in chocolate, labels it as "healthy and delicious," and sells it in a grocery store, it's still not real food. Got it?

When eating clean food, we are eating closer to nature, with as few stops between us and the farm as possible. When eating clean, we are avoiding pretend foods that were invented in a lab, using ingredients we can't spell, and ultra-processed for our modern world. An apple doesn't need a label.

Clean foods include organic vegetables, fruit, nuts and seeds, healthy fats, and pastured animals. Clean foods are alive, with enzymes that make them break down in our tummies — or on the counter if we leave them out. In other words, they rot. That's a good sign. (Side note: I've got a McDonald's apple pie in my office that is over six years old. Kids still want to eat it, as it looks like the day I bought it. I also had some fries, but after three years, someone actually ate them because they didn't know. Oops.)

Eating clean food fuels our bodies and levels out our blood sugar, reduces inflammation, promotes muscle building and fat loss, balances hormones, heals the gut, and supports proper digestion and elimination.

Unfortunately, all that changes when we eat pretend food. Our health has suffered immensely since we stopped eating from our natural habitat. Modern health epidemics like cardiovascular disease, diabetes, cancer, high blood pressure, and atherosclerosis were not found in tribes like the Maya of Central America, the Arctic Inuit, and the Hadza in Africa, until pretend foods were introduced to them.

Food's Natural State

Avoiding pretend food is challenging to be sure. Processed foods are cheaper to make and cheaper to store. However, we are making up that price difference with our health.

When we are eating clean, we are eating food that can be eaten in its natural state. That doesn't mean it must be eaten in its natural state but that it can be eaten in its natural state. Let's face it, we might not want to eat our animal proteins raw (although I love my sashimi!), but we could.

Food that is cooked, frozen, dried, smoked, marinated, fermented, or prepared with other real food products would still be considered part of the Clean Food Diet. However, any substance that must be manipulated and processed in order to eat it would not.

Case in point: wheat. You cannot go to a field and grab a handful of wheat and eat it for lunch. Nature has designed wheat in such a way that it is impossible to eat. First, there is the spikey head of the plant that we can't put in our mouths. And even if we can get past that, there is the wheat kernel that is so hard, we cannot crack it with our teeth, let alone chew it. And even if we manage to swallow it, our systems are not able to digest it. The kernel would go through us and come out just like it went in. (I know you are thinking about the last time you ate corn on the cob — ha!)

If something cannot be eaten in its natural state, then a lot of processing has had to happen to make it edible, and thus it is not classified as Clean Food. Clean Food's natural state also refers to food that does not contain GMOs, pesticides, and other toxins used to grow it, color it, or preserve it.

Foods with GMOs (genetically modified organisms) have been linked to infertility and cancer. A Russian study found that feeding hamsters GMOs led to complete sterility after only two or three generations. Similarly, glyphosates (a popular herbicide used on crops) have been studied extensively. Leading researcher Dr. N.L. Swanson found them to be disruptors to the human endocrine system, resulting in infertility, birth defects, miscarriage, and sexual dysfunction.

It's All in Your Mind

Diet behaviors like counting calories, weighing and measuring foods, going hungry, getting on the scale, and fixating on what you are not allowed to eat will make you a crazy person. And I would know; I was one. The key to success with Clean Food is to focus on what you want and move away from what you don't want.

What you want to eat is the highest quality veggies, fruits, proteins, and fats you can get your hands on. When you take a look at the Clean Food Diet List, you'll notice that there are a lot of things to eat! And they are incredibly delicious! These foods will help nourish your body to provide energy, reduce body fat, and decrease deadly inflammation.

What you want to stay away from are the pretend foods, which include sweets, grains and grain products, chips and snack foods, sports drinks and sodas. In short, you want to avoid sugar, empty carbs, and processed foods.

To get maximum results in the minimum amount of time with the Clean Food Diet, stay away from foods that are known to cause inflammation: legumes and dairy. Uh-oh, I just lost some of you. Don't worry, this does not mean that you can never have these foods again, as we will discuss a little later.

Now, you can obsess about rules and be a victim to them OR you can decide to take a more empowering position. Put yourself in a victim-free zone. Remember, choosing to eat clean is indeed, a choice. A choice you are making because . . . (Insert your own Big Why here).

The brain thinks in pictures, so use visualization to your advantage, not to your detriment. If you go to sleep counting donuts, or you walk by your favorite pizza lunch spot every day, your mind will continue to hold those images until you make them a reality. You cannot not think of something. (i.e. "Don't think of a pink elephant.") It's a matter of training yourself to focus on what you want, instead of what you don't want.

How to do that? Consistent practice. First, notice what you are thinking about (obsessing over). Instead of judging yourself and trying to not think about it anymore, replace that mental image with a supportive one.

Along with that, you can also do a few tangible things that will help you train your brain. Keep your refrigerator full of all the fresh, clean food you can jam in there, so that every time you open it, your brain sees you have so much delicious food to eat. Another idea is to make a vision board with all the clean foods you can eat, and/or the body shape you are working on, and/or a scuba diving trip you want to take. You can train your brain to eventually default to these empowering, healthful images and move you away from deprivation and crazy diet behaviors.

3 Ways to Do 21 Days

When you make a choice, you change the future.
-Deepak Chopra

If you're anything like me, you've tried lots of diets, and although they might have worked temporarily, they just haven't been successful in the long run. These experiences erode our confidence and unfortunately set us up for more failure.

Nothing propels success like success.

In biology, we witness how positive feedback systems work — the output enhances the original stimulus. The same thing happens in physics, where we find that a body in motion stays in motion. Psychologically, it holds true that when we feel positive and successful, we are more positive and successful. Using this information to our advantage, it is important to start your Clean Food Diet in a way that you can experience success right away. The positive momentum will keep you going and carry you through the challenges as they arise.

That is why we don't want to bite off more than we can chew. (Err, quite literally.)

There are three ways to succeed on this Clean Food Diet journey, and choosing which path depends on where you are starting from.

Accepting where you are now, without judgment, is the first step in creating a new outcome.

Level 1: Beginner

If you currently order a lot of your food through a car window or eat from packages or containers, then the Beginner track is where you want to start. Perhaps you've never really tried eating healthier before, and you might even be a little freaked out at the thought of it. It's okay. You can begin the Clean Food Diet by taking some small, but very significant, steps that you can succeed at. You will still see results and start feeling better. Many of my students feel so good at the end of 21 days that they are inspired to continue on and even step it up to the next level.

Level 2: 80/20

Perhaps you want to be a healthy eater but find it challenging to avoid packaged, processed, and prepared foods completely. You want to "cheat" from your healthy eating, even though you know it will impact your results. You have the drive but not the discipline. This is fine. Most of my students are in this place when they begin and are pleasantly surprised when they notice their cravings start to disappear and their clothes feel a little looser.

Level 3: Clean KUT

Are you ready to focus on the best nutrition for your body? Have you tried a million diets, found limited success, but are willing to do whatever it takes to feel better? Are you ready to "kut" out the pretend foods and replace them with the whole, real, and clean foods your body needs? Or maybe you just know that eating well and nourishing your body will take your health to the next level. Well, Clean KUT is for you. Your best results will come fastest on this plan.

Choose the level that you know you can succeed at. I cannot stress this enough. After working with thousands of people, I have seen failure happen many times. Not because of the Clean Food Diet nutrition plan, but because enthusiasm for transformation is not enough.

Janet was really excited about changing her body. She had two friends who had lost a lot of unwanted pounds doing my program, and she was ready for her turn. She had gained a lot of weight when she was pregnant (ten years ago), had stopped taking care of herself when she went back to her corporate job (nine years ago), and had been experiencing bouts of depression since her mother passed (five years ago).

Janet ate a lot of her meals out and bought packaged foods to heat up at home for the family, but now she wanted to change. She wanted to jump right into Level 3 because she figured that would give her the fastest and most dramatic results. The first few days were hard but she did it. Then stress hit and some of her old cravings took over, and off the clean eating wagon she jumped, face first.

She felt terrible about herself, which made her eat more crap, which made her feel worse . . . and of course did not get the results she was looking for. It would have been much better if she had started at the Beginner Level and succeeded there first.

Choose the Level that suits you best: Beginner, 80/20, or Clean KUT. It's okay that you choose one that is challenging, but it also must be doable! Remember, success is the most important factor at the start of this journey. The ultimate goal is to set up new, supportive, clean eating habits that you can maintain for a lifetime. (What, you thought this was something that you only had to do for 21 days? Ha!)

Once you have decided, find the Clean Food Diet List in the Level you have chosen.

Make sure to eat three to six meals per day, determined by your hunger level. This means no less than three meals and no more than six meals (and/or snacks) per day, with at least two hours in between. You want to work towards the ideal of three satisfying meals, spaced throughout the day.

Eat what you like from the Clean Diet Food List for your meal until you feel satiated, not stuffed. Eat slower, notice how you are feeling, and give yourself permission to leave food on your plate when you have had enough.

What to Eat

Understandably, some of you are unfamiliar with what it feels like to eat enough and yet not too much. This could be due to a malfunction in your neurotransmitters from unbalanced hormones. Don't worry. Here is what each meal should consist of:

- As many organic vegetables as you can eat. Dr. Terry Wahl suggests we aim for nine cups per day. That's a lot of veggies but you can do it! (She had a very Big Why — to heal herself of Multiple Sclerosis. Check out her TED.talk.)
- A serving of healthy fat from you Clean Food Diet List that is approximately the size of your thumb.
- A serving of quality, pasture-raised protein the size of the palm of your hand.

The portion sizes are approximate — don't drive yourself crazy! Remember, eat until you are satisfied but not stuffed. If you get hungry between meals, you just need more fat or protein, so make adjustments accordingly.

What Not to Eat

For the next 21 days, stay away from all variants of:

1. Sugar — natural or artificial sweeteners added to sweet or savory food products.
2. Grains — wheat, barley, rye, rice, and corn, including pasta and bread.
3. Legumes — beans, including soy, soy products, and peanuts.
4. Dairy — milk, cheese, sour cream, etc.
5. Processed Foods — or anything including artificial ingredients.

Stick with the Level you have chosen for the entire 21 days. Make a commitment at the beginning and then just do it. I know it's tempting to take it day by day and to change your mind to suit your mood, but that's just not how you master your life.

Level Up

If you started at Beginner or at 80/20, and you have a Big Why, then it's time to level up. Doing Clean KUT for 21 days will give your gut the opportunity to heal, and you might be surprised at how great you feel. I can't tell you how many times I have heard, "I didn't know I wasn't feeling good until I felt great!"

Once you are feeling good and enjoying your ideal weight, the 80/20 plan is a fine maintenance program for you.

Preparing for Success

You will find the key to success under the alarm clock.
-Benjamin Franklin

Wishing for success and planning for success are two separate activities. One is passive and the other is very, very active. The only way to ensure success with the Clean Food Diet is to actively plan in advance, and it all starts with your calendar. Yes, you have to schedule your success. Let's start now.

Pull out your calendar and let's take a look at your week. You need to schedule time to:

1. Clean out your fridge and your cupboards. No joke. Anything that is not on your Clean Food List must leave the premises. You think those "healthy cookies" are important to keep in your pantry in case you have company, but they know your name and will call to you in the middle of the night. You should only have to do this once. While you're at it, get rid of that stuff hiding in your desk at work too.

2. Create meal plans, choose recipes, and make a shopping list. I've included three weeks' worth in this book, but you still need to make the time to read them over and prepare your lists. Please note that any additional snacks need to be added to the weekly shopping list. If you are starting from scratch, this activity could take one to two hours per week.

3. Grocery shopping. Nobody seems to want to write this down in their calendar — they think they are just going to squeeze it in after work or something. Nope. It's going to take some time and effort, so allot the attention it deserves, especially on your first shopping trip. Don't stress out, as you may be navigating through some new areas of your grocery store. Make sure to include travel time in your calendar.

4. Preparing groceries. When you get home with your groceries, you need to put them away, of course, but it is also a great time to wash and cut up some of your veggies, so they are available for easy and fast snacks and/or ready to use for meals.

5. Make your meal. What time are you going to eat each day? How long will it take to prepare that meal? Write it in your calendar. Personally, I don't like to cook every meal of every day, so I double up and make two plates of food at dinner and keep one for the morning's breakfast. Yumm.

6. Eat. You must wrap your head around the idea that you need to take time to eat. Sitting. Chewing. Enjoying. Digesting. Oh, and throw in an uplifting conversation with a friend or family in there for good measure.

If you don't have time to shop, cook, sit and eat your food, you don't have time for success. Period. In my experience, people don't have a weight problem, they have a time management problem.

Meal Planning

To be prepared is half the victory.
-Miguel de Cervantes

Later in this book are twenty-one days of menus, with recipes and weekly shopping lists for your convenience. I purposely chose recipes that might be new, in order to ignite your taste buds and open up fresh options for you. However, I know that sometimes these prepared menus and lists add more stress if they are too different from the way you currently use (or don't use) your kitchen.

I get asked for recipes all the time. The first question I ask in return is, "How often do you currently use a recipe?" Or better yet, "When was the last time you used a recipe to make dinner?" You see, most people do not use recipes. Most of us have a repertoire of about three to five meals that we make on a regular basis. What are yours? Write them down. These are typically a few of your favorite meals that you always have and you buy the ingredients in the store without even thinking about it. I call these your "GO TO" meals.

Success with your Clean Food Diet is all about establishing new clean GO TO meals and always having the ingredients in your house. For instance, on any given day you can go into my refrigerator and you will find salmon, eggs, kimchi, avocado, asparagus, and spinach.

I can whip up at least three of my favorite meals with those ingredients, and so they are always in stock.

When you look at your current GO TO meals, are they using only the foods on your Clean Food List? If not, a good success strategy is to replace those meals with a clean version. If you love burgers and they are one of your GO TO meals, simply grill your burger and put it on your favorite salad instead of the dough ball you were eating it on last week. Your gut will thank you.

Don't be worried about eating the same thing all the time. Every meal does not have to be unique. Once you have gained confidence with the Clean Food Diet List you are working with, you will naturally try new things when you are ready.

Here are some fast and easy meals ideas that you can work with that don't really require the measuring and prep needed for most recipes.

Breakfast Ideas

- Scrambled eggs and bacon or sausage (add spinach for more deliciousness and fiber)
- Veggie omelet or frittata (quiche without the crust) with salad
- Banana pancakes (1 egg and 1 banana mixed with a fork and fried)
- Green protein smoothie (Clean KUT protein powder blended with water and your favorite green veggies)
- Smoked salmon with scrambled eggs, onions, capers
- Sweet potato hash with sausage and kale and mushrooms (fry it all up together!)
- Leftovers (my favorite)

Lunch

- Salad with chicken, fish, pork, beef, or lamb on top

- Soup (homemade is best)

- Lettuce wrap for burger, sausage, chicken skewers, etc.

- Beanless chili (ground meat with tomatoes, onion, garlic, and chili powder)

- Leftovers

Dinner

- Roast chicken, beef, lamb, and veggies on salad

- Stew on cauliflower rice (grated raw cauliflower)

- Meatballs or meatloaf with roasted veggies

- Grilled steak or fish with sweet potato fries and veggies

- Pulled pork or chicken or beef (slow cooker) with veggies

- Ground meat patties (beef, turkey, lamb) with grilled veggies

Grab-and-Go Snacks

- Eggs: hardboiled, deviled or egg muffins (what's that? Scramble eggs, pour into greased muffin tins and bake. Easy.)

- Coconut flakes

- Meat: drumsticks, meatballs, deli, jerky (read your ingredients!)
- Avocado (try drizzling some slices with balsamic vinegar!)
- Veggies: sticks with mustard, homemade mayo, almond butter, salsa, or guacamole
- Olives
- Nori
- Pickles and sauerkraut
- Can of fish
- Leftovers

Snackalicious

Did you know that snacking is a fairly new phenomenon? In fact, the word itself hasn't been part of the popular vernacular for even 50 years. Is "snack" a noun, verb, or adjective? All of the above, of course, because we love the word — and we love to snack.

Our brains think in pictures, and when the word "snack" comes up, we conjure lots of snack images, many of which are probably not on our Clean Food plan. With that in mind, let's redefine what a snack is.

A snack is a smaller meal. It is anything you would normally eat for a meal but perhaps a little smaller portion (or not). That's it, okay? If you're hungry between meals, have a little bit of real food.

That's a snack. You can also call it a meal. Easy.

This brings up another new word: grazing. Grazing is term used for non-stop eating. Although I have met a couple of people over the years that have found this to be a workable strategy, for most people it is not. Digestion is an important element of nourishment and we must give time for our bodies to complete this task and then rest. As a guideline, it is recommended to wait a couple of hours after a meal before eating again, in order to give your body a chance to digest what you have just eaten.

Bottom line? Eat when you are hungry but not too much. Then avoid eating again until your next meal. However, if you are hungry, wait at least two hours and then have a small meal (snack) to tide you over. Eventually your body will become a fat burner so you will be able to go longer between meals without getting hungry. Yeah!

"But I Can't Cook!"

I hear it a lot: "I don't know how to cook," or "I'm terrible in the kitchen," or my favorite, "I don't have time to cook!" If you say it, it must be true. But is that really what you want to be right about?

To manifest different results, you've got to do something different. You've got to make another way. And your way to clean eating and greater health is by making your own food. You can do it.

"Keep It Simple, Sweetie" is the new mantra. You don't need a bunch of fancy new recipes, you simply need the willingness to take the time to just do it. Here are my best tips on keeping things simple in the kitchen.

1.   Grill, roast, or sauté.

If you can do one of these, you are set. If not, then here is your first cooking lesson. Ready? Get out a fry pan and preheat it with a little fat (coconut oil is delish) to coat the bottom, so your food won't stick. Then put in your veggies or your protein. Sprinkle with a little sea salt and fresh pepper. Turn over or stir until done. Put it on a plate and eat it. Good job. Seriously, it is not any more difficult than that.

2.   Cook more to have leftovers.

Whenever you cook, make more than what you will eat in one meal. Leftovers are healthy, delicious, and faster than the local drive-thru restaurant. Sometimes I cook something that I'm not even having for dinner, but it will make another meal faster. For example, if I am roasting veggies in the oven for dinner, I add another roasting pan with sweet potatoes on it. I save those for tomorrow. They are easy to mash or just reheat in the microwave and it saves me the half hour they take in the oven.

3.   Consistency is better than variety.

Don't worry about eating the same thing all the time, as long as it is on your Clean Food List. Let's face it, up until now you have not been eating something different for every meal of the week, so it's unreasonable to think that when you start eating clean, you should. Trust that as you feel more confident and are able to take more time, you will eventually venture out and try new things.

4.   Have fun.

A good attitude in the kitchen goes a long way, so do what you need to do to make it fun. Your food will taste better with a cup of good vibes, so crank up the music or have a friend or family member join you. Keep things simple and, remember, you can't fail. If something doesn't taste good, just prepare something else. No biggy!

Clean Food Lists

We like lists because we don't want to die.
-Umberto Eco

Okay, it's time to get down to brass tacks, or rather, the meat and potatoes (ahem) of the Clean Food Diet. Although there might be some foods on the lists you have never heard of before, it doesn't mean you have to eat them. Just as there might be some foods that are inadvertently missing. These lists are meant for reference and to get your creative juices (and salivary glands) flowing.

NOTE: For your convenience, the CFD Food List is available as a free download at www.MasterMel.com/CFD

Vegetables

Veggies are the backbone of a Clean Food Diet. Aim for nine cups a day! There are many delicious ways to prepare your veggies:

- Raw — salad or chopped (with guacamole, yumm!)
- Grilled — coat with a little olive oil, salt, and pepper
- Roasted in the oven — coat with a little olive oil, salt, and pepper
- Steamed — cooked with the steam of boiling water
- Blanched — briefly dropped in boiling water and then taken out before cooking begins
- Sautéed — in butter, ghee, or coconut oil

Mastery Tips:

- Buy organic whenever possible. A great reference is the Environmental Working Group's guide (ewg.org), which identifies the most chemically laden, conventionally grown fruits and veggies, known as the "Dirty Dozen," along with the "Clean Fifteen."

- Buy fresh, and don't overcook

- Bring out the natural flavor of veggies by squeezing fresh lemon on them before serving

- Make your own salad dressing!!!

Sulfur Rich Veggies

Artichoke
Asparagus
Bok Choy
Broccoli
Brussel Sprouts
Cabbage (all)
Cauliflower
Celery
Garlic
Onions
Jicama
Leeks
Mushrooms
Radish
Shallots

Greens

Arugula
Chicory
Collard Greens
Dandelion
Endive
Kale
Lettuce (all)
Mustard Greens
Spinach
Swiss Chard
Turnip Greens
Watercress

Sea Vegetables

Seaweed/Nori
Dulse
Hijiki
Kombu
Laver
Wakame

Fruit Veggies

Cactus
Chilis
Cucumber
Eggplant
Okra
Olives
Peppers
Squash
Tomatillos
Tomato
Zucchini

Sprouts

Alfalfa Sprouts
Broccoli Sprouts
Fenugreek
Onion Sprouts
Sunflower Sprouts

Protein

Animal proteins contain all the essential amino acids our bodies need, along with many minerals and vitamins that are efficient and easy to absorb. But what about our vegetarian friends? We'll discuss more about that later. Meanwhile, here are some animal food choices. Remember, it's more about quality than quantity when it comes to protein.

There are several clean ways to cook protein but my favorites are slow cooking and grilling.

Mastery Tips:

- Choose wild when possible.
- Choose free-range, grass-fed or "pastured" (not pasteurized — that's something completely different) whenever possible.
- Get to know your farmer. Find suppliers from sustainable farms who treat their animals humanely, without antibiotics, growth hormones, and other drugs.
- Don't overcook as it tends to lose its flavor and get hard or rubbery.
- Season with quality sea salt and freshly ground pepper.
- Searing your protein at a high temperature will lock in juices. You will know it is ready to turn over in the pan when it no longer sticks.

Beef

Ground
Ribs
Roast
Steak
Tongue
Tri tip

Pork

Bacon
Chops
Ham
Loin
Roast
Shoulder

Shellfish

Clam
Crab
Lobster
Mussels
Oysters
Roe
Scallops
Sea Urchin
Shrimp

Fish

Bass
Cod
Flounder
Halibut
Mackerel
Mahi Mahi
Perch
Salmon
Sardines
Snapper
Tilapia
Trout
Tuna

Poultry

(Chicken, Turkey, Quail, Hen, etc.)
Breasts
Drumsticks
Ground
Thigh
Whole Roasted
Wings

Lamb

Chop
Rack
Roast

Exotics Other

Bison
Goat
Rabbit
Ostrich
Frog
Snake
Venison

Other

Eggs – Omega 3
Protein Powder
Organ Meats
(heart, liver, kidney, etc.)

Fat

Quality fats are where it's at. We need fat for energy, to produce important hormones, absorb vitamins, keep us warm, curb our hunger, and conduct nerve impulses to and from the brain. Besides that, fat makes other food taste even more delicious.

Mastery Tips:

- Select oils that are organic, extra virgin, and/or unrefined.

- Nuts and seeds need to be raw in order to provide quality fat.

- If it smells bad, don't eat it. Oils can be very sensitive and can go rancid. That goes for nuts and seeds as well.

- Don't go nuts for nuts. Although they are a good source of Omega-3 fats, many nuts also have inflammatory Omega-6 fats, so no more than a small handful per day. Or none.

Oils

Avocado Oil
Coconut Oil
Duck Fat
Flaxseed Oil
Hazelnut Oil
Lard (Pork Fat)
Macadamia Oil
Olive Oil
Palm Oil (Unrefined)
Pistachio Oil
Sesame Oil
Walnut Oil
Tallow (Beef Fat)

Foods

Avocado
Butter (grass-fed)
Coconut Butter
Coconut Milk
Ghee (grass-fed)

Nuts & Seeds

Acorn Squash Seeds
Almonds
Brazil Nuts
Cashews
Chestnuts
Chia Seeds
Flax Seeds
Hazelnuts
Hemp Seeds
Kabocha Seeds
Macademia Nuts
Pecans
Pine Nuts
Pistachios
Pumpkin Seeds
Sunflower Seeds
Walnuts

Fruit

Although there is nothing in fruit that your body can't get from veggies and meat, it is a delectable treat and should be treated as such. Enjoy it as a whole food in addition to your meal, not a substitute for other foods, and beware, the more sugar you consume, the more sugar you will crave.

Mastery Tips:

- Buy local and in season for best nutritional value

- Eat a variety of fruits that are in season

- Choose organic whenever possible. (see EWG's guide)

- If fat loss is your goal, limit fruit to one serving per day.

Least Sugar	Moderate Sugar	Most Sugar
Apricots	Apple	Banana
Blackberries	Grapefruit	Guava
Blueberries	Grapes	Mangos
Cherries	Lychee	Melons
Figs	Orange	Papaya
Grapefruit	Passion	Pineapple
Kiwi	Pear	
Nectarine		
Peach		
Plums		
Raspberries		
Strawberries		

Spices and Seasonings

Spice up your meal by trying different herbs and spices to add a new twist to your favorite veggies or proteins.

Mastery Tips:

- Those old spice jars in your cupboard that you've had for five years are not going to make your food taste better. Stop it.

- Dried seasonings are great but venture out and try some fresh herbs too.

- Avoid prepackaged seasoning packages (read your labels!)

Allspice	Cumin	Paprika
Anise	Curry	Parsley
Basil	Dill	Peppercorns
Bay Leaves	Fennel Seed	Peppermint
Black Pepper	Garlic Powder	Poppy seed
Bragg's Aminos	Garlic Salt	Rosemary
Caraway Seed	Ginger	Saffron
Cardamom	Lavender	Sage
Cayenne Pepper	Lemon Grass	Sea Salt
Celery Seed	Lemon Pepper	Sesame Seed
Chili Pepper	Mint	Spearmint
Cilantro	Mustard	Tarragon
Cinnamon	Mustard Seeds	Thyme
Cloves	Nutmeg	Tumeric
Coconut Aminos	Onion Seed	Vanilla
Coriander	Oregano	

Starches

Avoiding grains is easier when you replace them with delicious and nutritious sweet potatoes in moderation. The following carbohydrates are low on the glycemic index (measuring sugar impact), yet high in fiber, minerals, vitamins, and antioxidants. Roast them, mash them, or sauté them in coconut oil.

Mastery Tips:

- The body does not need starches, so don't eat them if you are not interested.

- Eat them in addition to veggies and protein, not instead of.

- The amount you consume should be in proportion to your activity level and fitness goals. For instance, as a carb, they are not great for weight loss but are awesome for recovery after a hard workout.

Plantain
Sweet Potato
Tapioca
Taro
Yams

Beverages

You need water. Nothing replaces it but if you want some of these other drinks, help yourself.

Mastery Tips:

- Not all kombucha is created equal. Look for raw and organic.
- Almond milk has become more commercially available, so read your labels. It should only have one ingredient other than water — almonds. It is super easy to make your own.
- Coconut milk is hard to get fresh, so canned is fine. Again, read your labels!

Almond Milk
Carbonated Water
Coconut Milk
Coconut Water
Coffee
Kombucha
Tea
Water

The Plan

Our goals can only be reached through a vehicle of a plan, in which we must
fervently believe, and upon which we must vigorously act.
There is no other route to success.
-Pablo Picasso

In the last chapter, you got to see all the delicious food included in the Clean Food Diet. Now it's time to put it all together in a plan.

In the next chapter you'll find a 21-day Clean Food Diet Guide with menus, recipes, and shopping lists to make it super easy for you to follow. If you would like to design your own menus, here are the four Clean Food Diet guidelines to help you plan your daily meals.

1. Every meal and/or snack consists of: veggies, protein, and a healthy fat.
2. Fruit is eaten according to your personal goals.
3. Eat a minimum of three times per day, maximum six.
4. Leave at least two hours between meals and snacks.

Portion Sizes

The quantity of food that you consume is adjustable to how hungry you are. The idea is to avoid diet behaviors like counting calories or weighing and measuring food and instead, eat what you want from your Clean Food Diet list until you are satisfied but not stuffed. When you are hungry and require more fuel, you will eat more; when you are not, you won't.

With that in mind, many students I work with still want to know what a "normal" portion size is. *Okay, okay.*

There are many detailed formulas out there as to how much food you need based on how much muscle mass you carry, but I prefer the simple eyeball method and offer up these approximate portion sizes.

Veggies – Aim for 9 cups a day! (A handful is a cup)

Healthy Fats – 1 tablespoon per meal (size of your thumb)

Protein – 4 to 8 oz. per meal (size of the palm of your hand)

Fruit – 1 to 3 servings a day, based on your goals

Now I know you are wondering, *what's all this hoopla about fruit? Isn't fruit full of the wonderful nutrients that a body loves?* Yes, it is. But fruit is also full of sugar. In an earlier chapter, we talked about how our bodies cannot burn sugar and fat at the same time, so if your goal is to burn more body fat, you will want to avoid copious amounts of fruit.

Mastery Tips

- Drink water before a meal, not during. Beverages water down your digestive enzymes, making them less effective.

- Enjoy your food and eat slowly. Your digestion cycle starts when you first see and smell your food.

- Chew your food. You can't absorb nutrients from food that does not digest.

- Leaving time between meals gives your body time to digest and rest.

- If you can, eat after your workout (not right before), when your muscles are looking to replenish glucose stores.

The Clean Food Diet Levels

Below is a handy grid of the foods that are included on each level of the Clean Food Diet.

Grid key:

Yes – means it's included

No – it's not included

Mod – to be eaten in moderation (1-2 times per week)

Veg – this is the Clean KUT level for vegetarians

NOTE: For your convenience, the CFD Levels grid is available as a free download at: www.MasterMel.com/CFD

VEGGIES	Beg	80/20	Clean
Cooked, raw or fermented	yes	yes	yes

PROTEIN	Beg	80/20	Clean
Bone broth - homemade	yes	yes	yes
Eggs	yes	yes	yes
Meat and poultry	yes	yes	yes
Organ meats	yes	yes	yes
Seafood	yes	yes	yes
Protein powder - read labels!	yes	yes	mod
Processed meat – sausage, bacon, salami, jerky	yes	yes	mod
Preseasoned meats	no	no	no

FATS	Beg	80/20	Clean
Animal fat – lard, tallow, duck	yes	yes	yes
Avocados	yes	yes	yes
Avocado oil	yes	yes	yes
Coconut – oil, butter, cream, meat, milk	yes	yes	yes
Ghee	yes	yes	yes
Nut oils - macadamia, etc.	yes	yes	yes
Olives & olive oil – extra virgin	yes	yes	yes
Palm kernel oil, red palm oil	yes	yes	yes
Raw nuts and seeds	yes	yes	mod
Butter	yes	yes	no
Industrial oils - seed & vegetable oils like corn, soy, canola, etc.	no	no	no

FRUITS	Beg	80/20	Clean
Low sugar- berries, plums peaches etc.	yes	yes	mod
High sugar- tropicals, bananas, apples, etc.	yes	mod	no
Dried fruit, fruit juice	no	no	no
Soda or sports drinks	no	no	no

DAIRY	Beg	80/20	Clean	Veg
Ghee (clarified butter)	yes	yes	yes	yes
Butter (grass-fed)	yes	yes	no	no
Fermented dairy	yes	yes	no	no
Hard cheese (as seasoning)	yes	yes	no	no
Goat/sheep cheese	yes	mod	no	no
Full-fat cream	yes	mod	no	no
Raw dairy products	yes	mod	no	no
All other pasteurized dairy	no	no	no	no

LEGUMES	Beg	80/20	Clean	Veg
Green beans, sugar peas and snap peas	yes	yes	mod	yes
Fermented soy	yes	mod	mod	yes
Beans - adzuki, black, broad, garbonzo, pinto, white, kidney	yes	mod	no	yes
Lentils, split pea	yes	mod	no	yes
Peanuts	no	no	no	no
Soy - tofu, edamame, etc.	no	no	no	no

GRAINS & STARCHES	Beg	80/20	Clean	Veg
Plantains	yes	yes	yes	yes
Sweet potatoes	yes	yes	yes	yes
Tapioca	yes	yes	yes	yes
Taro	yes	yes	yes	yes
Yams	yes	yes	yes	yes
Sprouted &/or fermented grains	yes	yes	mod	yes
Buckwheat	yes	yes	no	yes
Wild rice	yes	yes	no	yes
White rice	yes	yes	no	yes
Corn	yes	mod	no	no
Amaranth	yes	no	no	yes
Brown rice	yes	no	no	yes
Oats	yes	no	no	no
Quinoa	yes	no	no	yes
Potatoes – white, yellow, purple	mod	mod	no	no
Bread	no	no	no	no
Pasta	no	no	no	no
Wheat, barley, rye	no	no	no	no

SEASONINGS	Beg	80/20	Clean
Fresh herbs and spices	yes	yes	yes
Mustard (no sugar)	yes	yes	yes
Sea salt	yes	yes	yes
Spices	yes	yes	yes
Coconut/Bragg's aminos	yes	yes	yes
Commercial spreads & sauces (incl. ketchup)	yes	no	no
MSG	no	no	no
Packaged seasonings	no	no	no
Soy sauce, tamari	no	no	no

BEVERAGES	Beg	80/20	Clean
Carbonated water	yes	yes	yes
Coconut milk/water	yes	yes	yes
Lemon or lime juice	yes	yes	yes
Coffee and tea (caff)	yes	mod	mod
Vegetable juice	yes	mod	no
Almond milk, rice milk	yes	no	no
Fruit juice, smoothies or "natural" drinks	no	no	no
Milk – (see DAIRY)	no	no	no
Soy milk	no	no	no
Soda or sports drinks	no	no	no

ALCOHOL	Beg	80/20	Clean
Kombucha	yes	yes	yes
Cooking with alcohol	yes	yes	no
Vodka, tequila or wine	1x/day	1x/wk	no
Other spirits	1x/day	no	no

SWEETS	Beg	80/20	Clean
Chocolate 70%+	yes	yes	no
Natural sugars: coconut sugar, maple syrup, honey, molasses	yes	yes	no
Stevia	yes	yes	no
Sugar in savory foods	yes	no	no
Xylitol	yes	no	no
All other sugar or artificial sweeteners	no	no	no

Clean Food Diet 21-Day Guide

Never eat more than you can lift.
-Miss Piggy

I hope you enjoy the menus and recipes included here. You can follow each day to the letter, pick and choose what you like, or simply use it as a guide to inspire your own creative impulses to make clean, delicious meals.
Bon Appetit!

Week One

Week 1 Menus

Monday
Breakfast: Breakfast Salad
Lunch: Curried Chicken Salad
Dinner: Seared Tuna with Roasted Bok Choy & Cucumber-Tomato Salad

Tuesday
Breakfast: Soft-Boiled Eggs with Smoked Salmon and Bok Choy
Lunch: Tuna Niçoise Salad
Dinner: Steak with Mushrooms and Garlic Cauliflower Rice

Wednesday
Breakfast: Cauliflower Porridge with Berries and Walnuts
Lunch: Steak Salad
Dinner: Carrot Ginger Soup and Lemon Chicken Skewers

Thursday

Breakfast: Overnight Chia Seed Pudding with Berries and Nuts

Lunch: Carrot Soup with Chicken on Salad

Dinner: Spaghetti Squash with Meatballs

Friday

Breakfast: Chia Seed Pudding

Lunch: Leftover Squash with Meatballs

Dinner: Rosemary Chicken with Sweet Potatoes and Broccoli

Saturday

Breakfast: Herb Omelet with Bacon

Lunch: Chicken Salad

Dinner: Salmon with Mashed Sweet Potato and Simple Salad

Sunday

Breakfast: Kitchen Sink Frittata

Lunch: Curried Salmon Lettuce Wraps

Dinner: Beef Stew

Week 1 Recipes

Breakfast Salad

This is a quick, high-fat (the good kind), and high-protein breakfast that keeps you going all the way until lunchtime. This is my go-to breakfast on weekdays when I don't have a lot of time but need something filling.

2 cups arugula (or your favorite mixed greens)
½ avocado, sliced
¾ cup smoked salmon (or a different protein leftover)
1 tablespoon olive oil
½ juiced lemon
2 eggs
Ghee or other healthy fat for cooking
Salt and pepper to taste

In a bowl, place a handful of arugula, ½ sliced avocado, and 3 to 4 pieces of smoked salmon broken into bite-size chunks. Drizzle 1 tablespoon olive oil, ½ juiced lemon, and salt and pepper to taste. Mix and set on a plate. Cayenne or pepper flakes are a great addition if you like a kick.

Prepare 2 free-range organic eggs however you like them best. Cook your eggs in ghee, beef tallow, or leftover bacon grease. If you are frying eggs, keep the heat low, so the white does not become rubbery.

Place eggs over the salad and enjoy.

Curried Chicken Salad

This is a great desk lunch or lunch on the go. It can be made with either leftover chicken or canned chicken and can be eaten straight or made into a lettuce wrap. Apples are a great addition if you choose.

1 can organic chicken in water

1 large carrot, grated

1 stalk celery, chopped into ¼ inch pieces

¼ cup walnuts, chopped

1 handful arugula (or kale if you are making it a day ahead as it keeps longer)

½ bunch parsley, chopped

1-2 garlic cloves, minced

½ juiced lemon

2 tablespoons olive oil

1 teaspoon paprika

½ teaspoon curry powder

Pinch of cayenne if you like it spicy

Salt and pepper to taste

Drain chicken and place in a bowl. Add the carrots, celery, walnuts, arugula, parsley, and garlic. Mix well.

Add the lemon juice, olive oil, and all spices. Taste and adjust to your palate.

Either eat immediately or place into a container.

Seared Tuna with Roasted Bok Choy and Cucumber-Tomato Salad

1 lb. tuna steaks

4 garlic cloves, minced

2 inches ginger, grated or minced

3 tablespoons toasted sesame oil

1 large cucumber, peeled and sliced

1 pkg. cherry tomatoes, halved

½ red onion, thinly sliced and soaked in ¼ cup rice vinegar for 5 minutes

3 limes, 2 juiced and 1 sliced into quarters for serving

1 bunch scallions, thinly sliced

3 bunches bok choy, ends cut off and leaves separated

2 tablespoons sesame seeds

Coconut oil or ghee for cooking

2 tablespoons miso paste (or tahini)

Salt and pepper to taste

Preheat oven to 400°.

In a bowl combine ½ of the minced garlic and ½ of the minced ginger, 1 tablespoon sesame oil and paste. Rub marinade on tuna steaks and let sit for at least 20 minutes on the counter.

Meanwhile, combine cucumbers, tomatoes, and onions with the vinegar. Pour in half the lime juice, 1 tablespoon sesame oil, half the scallions, and salt and pepper to taste.

In a large bowl, mix the remaining garlic, ginger, miso paste, sesame oil, scallions, and sesame seeds. Mix in the bok choy and make sure it is thoroughly coated.

Place bok choy on a sheet tray and cook in the oven for twelve minutes.

Heat a skillet on medium-high (non-stick or cast iron is preferred, so the fish does not stick to the pan). Place a little coconut oil or ghee in the pan. Once the pan is hot, place fish in the pan and sear for 3 minutes on either side.

Remove bok choy from the oven and put some on the plate, scoop a portion of the cucumber salad next to it, and top with the seared tuna. Place a slice of lime on each plate to use on the tuna. Enjoy!

Soft-Boiled Eggs with Smoked Salmon and Bok Choy

4 eggs
1 tablespoon olive oil or ghee
½ red onion, sliced
Leftover bok choy, chopped into bite-size pieces
3 pieces smoked salmon, broken into smaller chunks

Place eggs in a pot of water with salt. Bring to a boil and then turn off heat. Allow to sit in the water for 8 minutes if you like soft boiled, 10 for medium, or 12 for hard.

Heat a pan on medium heat. Once hot, put oil in the pan. Sauté the onions until translucent, then add bok choy and smoked salmon. Salt and pepper to taste.

Place veggie and salmon mixture on a plate and top with 2 peeled eggs.

Tuna Niçoise Salad

Can be made with leftover tuna or canned tuna and is quick and easy if you have boiled eggs leftover from breakfast.

Leftover tuna or 1 can tuna in water
½ container cherry tomatoes, halved
1 cup green beans, raw or blanched and sliced in half
2 boiled eggs, peeled and halved
½ cup niçoise olives, chopped
½ bunch chives, chopped
½ bunch parsley, chopped
Large handful baby kale or preferred green

Dressing:
1 tablespoon capers, chopped
1 juiced lemon
1 tablespoon olive oil
1 tablespoon Dijon mustard
2 anchovies, minced (optional but high in omega 3's)
1 pinch red pepper flake
Salt and pepper to taste

In a small bowl, combine all dressing ingredients and mix well. In a large bowl, combine all salad ingredients except eggs and then mix in dressing. Place the salad in a bowl and top with sliced eggs.

Steak with Mushrooms and Garlic Cauliflower Rice

2 steaks*, 1 is for dinner and 1 for next day's lunch
¼ cup ghee or other healthy fat (olive oil or beef tallow work well with this dish)
1 large yellow onion, thinly sliced
1 lb. of your favorite mushrooms, sliced (I love shitake)
5 garlic cloves, minced
¼ cup balsamic vinegar
½ bunch parsley, chopped
1 head cauliflower, grated
Salt and pepper to taste

*Choose whatever steak you like best. Rib eye is great for a big occasions or skirt steak for every day.

Preheat oven to 350°.

Season the steaks with sea salt and black pepper. Heat a skillet (preferably cast iron) on high heat. Place 2 tablespoons ghee or oil in the pan and get it hot. Place steaks on the pan and sear until dark golden brown. Flip over and brown on the other side. Place cast iron in the oven and for every half inch of thickness, cook for 5 minutes (for medium rare).

While the steak is cooking, heat another pan on medium-high heat. Put remaining ghee or oil into the pan and once hot, add the onions. Salt lightly and stir. Once translucent, add the mushrooms. When the mushrooms soften, add half the minced garlic. Stir until garlic becomes aromatic.

Pour in the balsamic vinegar and reduce until thickened slightly. Add ½ the parsley and fresh ground pepper.

Remove the steak from the oven and let it rest for 5 minutes before slicing across the grain.

While the steak rests, heat fat and stir in ½ of the minced garlic and add ⅔ of the cauliflower and the rest of the chopped parsley. (Put ⅓ cauliflower aside, unseasoned, for breakfast porridge tomorrow).

Place the garlic cauliflower rice on a plate, top with the sliced steak and then finished with the balsamic glazed mushroom and onions.

Cauliflower Porridge with Berries and Walnuts

A great way to use leftover cauliflower rice and get that morning cereal fix!

2 cups unseasoned cauliflower, grated
1 can coconut cream, well shaken
1 teaspoon cinnamon
1 teaspoon vanilla
1 tablespoon ginger, grated
1 cup mixed berries
½ cup walnuts, chopped

Combine cauliflower and ⅔ can coconut cream in a small pot on low heat. Add in cinnamon, vanilla, and ginger. Stir slowly until hot.

Place into a bowl and top with berries and nuts.

Steak Salad

1 steak, sliced

3 handfuls of your favorite greens (kale, arugula, or spinach work well)

Leftover mushrooms and onions

1 avocado, cubed

1 juiced lemon

2 tablespoons olive oil

1 tablespoon Dijon mustard

1 tablespoon vinegar of your choice

Salt and pepper to taste

In a large bowl, place salad greens, mushrooms, onions, and avocado.

In a small bowl, combine lemon juice, olive oil, mustard, vinegar, and salt and pepper.

Dress salad with salad dressing, or put into a little container to dress later.

Place steak on top. Enjoy!

Carrot Ginger Soup

6 large carrots, peeled and chopped into ½-inch-thick pieces

2 yellow onions, sliced

3 stalks celery, chopped into thick pieces

5 garlic cloves, peeled and smashed

2 inch-long pieces of ginger, chopped into 5 pieces

1 bunch scallions, chopped, green part separated

1 tablespoon curry powder

¼ cup coconut oil

1 container chicken or vegetable stock

¼ cup miso paste (or tahini)

1 can coconut milk

2 juiced limes

Salt and pepper to taste

Preheat oven to 375° and chop veggies.

In a large bowl, place veggies, garlic, ginger, white part of the scallions, curry powder, salt and pepper. Coat with melted coconut oil.

Place on a large parchment-lined baking sheet. Roast for 30 minutes, or until carrots are done.

In a blender put ⅓ of the mixture in at a time with enough stock to cover the vegetables. Blend until smooth and pour into a pot. Blend in paste, can of coconut milk, and lime juice. Add more stock to reach desired thickness. Once the soup is hot, place in a bowl, and top with chopped green scallions.

Lemon Chicken Skewers

These can be marinated in advance.

1 lb. chicken tenders cut in ½-inch strips
2 tablespoons olive oil
2 tablespoons juiced lemon
1 tablespoon parsley or cilantro
1 garlic clove, minced
½ teaspoon paprika
¼ teaspoon cumin
Salt and cayenne to taste
Wooden skewers
Coconut oil for cooking

Place chicken strips in a glass dish.

In a small bowl, whisk other ingredients together. Pour marinade over chicken until well coated. Put in the fridge for 20 minutes.

Soak skewers in water for a minimum of 10 minutes.

Thread chicken strips on skewers. Heat coconut oil in skillet.

Cook chicken skewers in skillet a few minutes on each side and serve placed across the bowl of carrot soup.

Chia Seed Pudding with Berries and Nuts

This recipe needs to be made the night before, and it can last for 2 to 3 days in the fridge. Chia seeds are a massive source of omega-3's, fiber, and protein.

¾ cup chia seeds
3 cups almond milk
1 scoop vanilla Whey Clean protein powder (Clean KUT)
1 can coconut milk, well shaken
1 tablespoon vanilla
1 cup blueberries

Topping:
Blueberries
Almonds or other nuts of your choice

In a blender, place almond milk, protein powder, coconut milk, vanilla, and blueberries.

In a container, mix this liquid with the chia seeds. Refrigerate and stir occasionally. Allow to sit in the fridge overnight. (Minimum 2 hours.)

Top with berries and mixed nuts.

Making the pudding for multiple days is great for people who don't have a lot of time in the morning. It is very easy to put them in individual jars topped with berries for a quick grab-and-go breakfast that keeps you full for hours.

Salad Dressing

Lunch is leftover carrot soup. Add leftover chicken into soup or to a salad if you like. Here is a salad dressing that works great with everything.

2 juiced lemons
2 garlic cloves, minced
1 shallot, minced
¼ cup apple cider vinegar
2 tablespoons whole grain or Dijon mustard
¼ cup olive oil
Salt and pepper to taste

Place everything in a mason jar and shake vigorously. Can be used immediately or saved in the fridge for a week.

Spaghetti Squash with Meatballs

Spaghetti squash is a delicious and healthy vegetable, a good alternative to pasta, and kids love it too!

1 spaghetti squash, halved and seeded
1 lb. ground beef
½ lb. ground lamb (optional)
1 egg
¼ cup almond meal
4 garlic cloves, minced
1 teaspoon cumin
1 teaspoon paprika
2 teaspoons salt
1 teaspoon pepper
1 jar tomato sauce (sugar free)
1 bunch basil

Preheat oven to 375°.

Place spaghetti squash face down on a parchment-lined sheet tray. Place in the oven to roast. It will take about 45 minutes.

Meanwhile, in a large bowl, place ground meat, egg, almond meal, garlic, spices, salt, and pepper. Mix well with your hands.

Roll the meatball mixture into golf-ball-size rounds.

Heat a large skillet (cast iron is best) on medium-high heat and add in 2 tablespoons ghee or oil of your choice.

Place all of the meatballs in the pan and sear them for 4 minutes.

Pour the entire jar of tomato sauce into the pan. Shake pan lightly to get the sauce under the meatballs.

Place the pan in the oven and cook for 20 minutes.

Remove the squash and meatballs from the oven.

With a large spoon, scoop pasta-like squash out of the skin and into a bowls. Season with olive oil and salt and pepper to taste.

Place a scoop of squash in a bowl and top with a few meatballs and sauce. Add a little freshly chopped basil and dig in.

Leftover meatballs are great on a salad with balsamic vinegar and olive oil.

Rosemary Roasted Chicken with Sweet Potatoes and Broccoli

A whole chicken is great to use for days in different meals. Once you pick all the meat off the bones, you can make bone broth. Brining a chicken in vinegar and salt and pepper for at least 4 hours or up to 2 days in advance can tenderize it and add a lot of flavor.

1 large organic chicken
6 garlic cloves, minced
5 sprigs rosemary, chopped
3 tablespoons whole grain mustard
3 tablespoons ghee or olive oil
1 tablespoon salt
1 teaspoon pepper
1 yellow onion, sliced
2 lemons, halved
4 sweet potatoes
3 stalks broccoli
Salt and pepper to taste

Preheat oven to 350°.

In a small bowl, combine garlic, rosemary, whole grain mustard, ghee or oil, and about a tablespoon of salt and a teaspoon of pepper.

Rub marinade all over chicken.

In a large baking dish, lay chopped onions, lightly salted and peppered, and put chicken on top. Put lemon pieces inside the chicken.

Place chicken in the oven and roast for about an hour and a half, or until a thermometer inserted reads 165°.

Place the sweet potatoes on a parchment-lined sheet tray and place in the oven with the chicken. No need to peel. Cook until soft to the touch or a fork goes in really easy.

When you pull the chicken out of the oven, put a pot of water on to boil with 1 tablespoon of salt. Chop broccoli into bite-size florets. Flash boil for 4 minutes.

Put the chicken on a cutting board and pull the lemon out of the chicken. Squeeze juice of 1 lemon over it (careful, the lemons are hot).

Mix the broccoli, juice of the other lemon, and the grilled onions together in the baking dish.

The skin will pull easily away from the potatoes after they have sat out of the oven. Mash or cut up and drizzle with your favorite oil. Serve with cut up chicken and broccoli.

Herb Omelet with Bacon

Bacon is great in a million ways. Just make sure to get good organic, pastured bacon without nitrites. Also, save the bacon fat to use for cooking later.

6 strips of bacon

5 eggs

2 tablespoons water

½ cup of whatever herbs you have in the fridge (parsley, cilantro, chive, scallion, dill, etc.)

Salt and pepper to taste

Place bacon in a cold cast iron or non-stick pan. Turn on heat to medium and cook to your desired crispiness. Pour bacon fat into a mason jar to keep.

Crack eggs into a bowl, pour in 2 tablespoons water and all the herbs. Add a pinch of salt and pepper — and cayenne if you like it. Whisk well.

Use a tablespoon of bacon grease or olive oil and heat up a non-stick pan on medium heat.

Pour in egg mixture and stir gently. Allow to set slightly, and then mix again. Cover with a lid and allow to cook, turning the heat to low. Once the eggs are almost all the way cooked, use a spatula to fold the eggs in half. Turn off heat and cover for 2 minutes, allowing the inside to cook the rest of the way.

Serve with bacon on the side, or break the bacon up and put it in the middle of the omelet.

Chicken Salad

This salad is wonderfully versatile. Just about any meat and vegetable tastes great when made into a salad, as long as you have a good dressing.

Leftover chicken, chopped or shredded into bite-size pieces
Salad greens of your choice
Leftover broccoli

Pour your homemade salad dressing on the ingredients and mix until combined. Eat and enjoy.

Salmon, Sweet Potato, and Salad

Salmon is simple to cook and is full of all the right fat for your body. The roasted sweet potatoes from a previous dinner turn into an amazing mash the following day.

3 salmon filets, skin on is fine
Leftover sweet potato, mashed
1 lemon, halved
Olive oil and/or ghee
1 garlic clove, minced
Mixed greens
Salt and pepper to taste

Mix juice of ½ lemon and 1 tablespoon olive oil into the sweet potato mash. Place in a small pot to heat up when salmon is ready.

Heat a skillet to medium heat and add 1 tablespoon ghee or olive oil.

Place salmon skin side down and cook for about 4 minutes. Salt and pepper the top. Flip and cook for about 4 more minutes, or until it reaches desired doneness. I like it when the salmon is a little pink in the middle.

Turn off heat and flip back onto the skin side. Warm up the sweet potatoes.

Drizzle mixed greens with lemon and oil and serve with the sweet potatoes and salmon. Squeeze lemon over the salmon before eating.

Kitchen Sink Frittata

By the end of the week, the last straggling veggies and odds and ends of meat remain in the fridge. A frittata is a quick way to use up all of that to make breakfast for a crowd or to make an easy Monday.

6 eggs
Grilled veggies
Chicken or other meat, chopped
Herbs (any), chopped

Preheat oven to 325°.

In a large bowl, whisk the eggs and all other ingredients. Add salt and pepper.

Heat a non-stick pan with olive oil or ghee and pour in the egg mixture.

Put the skillet in the oven and cook until the mixture no longer jiggles when lightly shaken.

Curried Salmon Lettuce Wraps

This can easily be substituted with chicken.

Leftover salmon, broken up
1 carrot, grated
½ cucumber, peeled and thinly sliced
1 bunch scallions, chopped
1 bunch bib or red leaf lettuce (whichever has big enough leaves to fill)

Sauce:
1 juiced lime
2 tablespoons sesame oil
2 tablespoons rice vinegar
2 tablespoons miso paste (or tahini)
1 garlic clove, minced
1 teaspoon curry powder
1 teaspoon cumin

Mix all sauce ingredients together in a small bowl.

Using the lettuce as cups, fill with salmon, shredded carrot, and cucumber.

Drizzle sauce and sprinkle on scallions and enjoy.

Beef Stew

I use bone-in short rib so I can use the bones for bone broth afterward. A crock pot is really great for this recipe, but it can also be done in a covered baking dish.

5 bone-in short ribs
4 large carrots, peeled and cut into inch-thick pieces
2 bell peppers
1 large yellow onion, diced
8 garlic cloves, minced
1 tablespoon smoked paprika
1 tablespoon cumin
1 teaspoon thyme
¼ cup balsamic vinegar
1 container chicken or vegetable stock
Salt and pepper and cayenne to taste
1 bunch parsley, chopped

Preheat oven to 375°.

Coat the vegetables in the spices and a little oil. Roast them until under-done, about 20 minutes.

Salt and pepper the short ribs. Heat a skillet on high heat and brown the meat on all sides. Remove the meat from the pan and pour in the vinegar, scraping the bottom to get the flavor. Pour into a baking dish.

Place all the veggies and meat into the baking dish and pour in the stock until ingredients are half submerged. Cover with a tight-fitting lid.

Bake at 250° for 3 to 4 hours, depending on the size of the short ribs. Uncover and let cook for another 30 minutes. Serve in a bowl with fresh parsley sprinkled on top.

Week 1 Shopping List

Produce

2 large bags of organic carrots

1 bunch celery

6 large yellow onions

3 large cucumbers

4 heads garlic

3 bunches bok choy

1 head cauliflower

2 package cherry tomatoes

2 red onions

2 shallots

1 ginger root

14 lemons

6 limes

4 oranges

4 avocados

2 bell peppers

4 large sweet potatoes

1 large spaghetti squash

4 containers blueberries

2 containers blackberries

1 lb. mushrooms

3 bunches parsley

1 bunch basil

3 stalks broccoli

2 bunches cilantro

3 bunches scallions

1 large bunch arugula

1 large bunch baby kale

1 large head bib lettuce

1 small bunch rosemary

Meat, Eggs, Milk

1 qt. almond milk

2 dozen eggs

1 lb. tuna

3-4 filets salmon

1 large chicken

1 large chicken tenders (or breast)

5 bone-in short ribs

2 steaks

1 lb. ground beef

½ lb. ground lamb

1 pkg. bacon

1 can organic chicken in water

1 pkg. smoked salmon

Canned/Bottled Goods

1 large bottle cold-pressed virgin olive oil

1 large jar coconut oil

1 small bottle toasted sesame oil

1 jar ghee

1 jar tomato sauce

1 bottle apple cider vinegar

1 jar Dijon mustard

1 jar whole grain mustard

1 jar capers

1 container chicken or vegetable stock

3 cans coconut cream

1 can coconut milk

1 small jar anchovies (if you like them)

1 container miso paste (or jar of tahini)

Dry Goods and Spices

Smoked paprika

Paprika

Cumin

Red pepper flakes

Cayenne

Curry powder

Cinnamon

Vanilla

Sesame seeds

1 bag walnuts

1 bag sliced almonds

1 bag chia seeds

1 bag almond flour

Whey Clean Protein Powder (available at www.CleanKUT.com)

Week Two

Week 2 Menus

Monday
Breakfast: Over-Easy Egg with Garlicky Spinach
Lunch: Short Rib Lettuce Wraps
Dinner: Parchment Poached Fish with Braised Fennel

Tuesday
Breakfast: Overnight Chia Pudding
Lunch: Asian Fish Salad
Dinner: Beanless Chili with Salad (optional)

Wednesday
Breakfast: Overnight Chia Pudding
Lunch: Chili
Dinner: Beef and Broccoli

Thursday
Breakfast: Fried Eggs with Broccoli Beef
Lunch: Chili with a Side Salad
Dinner: Chicken Thighs with Herbed Cauliflower Rice and Green Sauce

Friday
Breakfast: Savory Cauliflower Porridge with Eggs and Green Sauce
Lunch: Chicken Salad with Green Goddess Dressing
Dinner: Pea Soup with Smoked Ham

Saturday

Breakfast: Protein Pancakes

Lunch: Pea Soup and a Simple Salad

Dinner: Chicken Fajitas and a Simple Salad

Sunday

Breakfast: Yam Hash with Fried Eggs

Lunch: Pea Soup or Kitchen Sink Salad

Dinner: Zucchini Noodles with Bolognese

Week 2 Recipes

Over-Easy Eggs with Garlicky Spinach

4 eggs

1 tablespoon olive oil

4 garlic cloves, minced

3 cups spinach

½ lemon

Salt and pepper to taste

Heat a small sauté pan on medium heat. Add half the olive oil. Sauté the garlic just until fragrant — be careful not to burn it. Add in the spinach, salt and pepper, and a squeeze of lemon, and cover with the heat off.

Heat a non-stick pan on medium heat, adding the remaining olive oil. Cook the eggs, flipping in the middle of the cooking process.

Put the spinach on the plate and top with the eggs and a sprinkle of salt and pepper.

Short Rib Lettuce Wraps

After the weekend, there's usually some meat leftover that you can use for lunch the following day. Shred it or slice it to use easily. If not, open a can of tuna or chicken.

Leftover short rib, shredded

Red leaf or bib lettuce, washed and separated

1 avocado, sliced

2 carrots, grated

½ bunch parsley, chopped

Fill lettuce cups with the shredded beef, and then top with avocado, carrots, and a little parsley.

Parchment Poached Fish with Braised Fennel

1 ½ lbs. (4 servings) sea bass or a white fish of your choice
2 cups baby kale or spinach
1 yellow onion, thinly sliced
3 fennel bulbs, halved and thinly sliced
2 zucchinis or summer squash
2 lemons, sliced into thin half circles
3 garlic cloves, minced
4 tablespoons olive oil
½ bunch parsley, chopped
Salt, pepper and cayenne to taste

Preheat oven to 300°. Salt, pepper, and cayenne the fish.

In a wide, shallow baking dish, layer the kale, onion, fennel, zucchini, and half the lemon slices. Sprinkle the garlic over the veggies along with 2 tablespoons olive oil. Season the veggies with salt, pepper, and cayenne if you want them to be spicy.

Lay the fish on top of the veggies and layer the remaining lemon slices over top the fish. Sprinkle ½ of the parsley over the entire dish. Drizzle the remaining 2 tablespoons of olive oil over the fish. Cover fish with parchment paper, and then cover entirely with tin foil, making sure it is sealed around the edges.

Bake for 30 minutes. Remove from oven and remove the cover. Check that the fish is cooked through and the veggies are lightly steamed. Use a spatula to serve the veggies and fish, and sprinkle each plate with a little bit of parsley.

Overnight Chia Pudding

This recipe needs to be made the night before. It can last for 3 days in the fridge. Spirulina or chlorella and maca are optional super foods that add to your overall health. Spirulina detoxes heavy metals, eliminates candida, is alkalizing, boosts energy, and is filled with vitamins and minerals. Maca is rich in vitamins B, C, and E, and provides plenty of calcium, zinc, iron, magnesium, phosphorous, and amino acids. It helps with sexual function, women's health, mood, energy levels, and skin.

¾ cup chia seeds

3 cups almond milk

1 scoop vanilla Whey Clean protein powder (Clean KUT)

1 can coconut milk, well shaken

1 tablespoon vanilla

1 tablespoon spirulina

1 tablespoon maca

1 cup blueberries

Topping:

Blueberries

Toasted almonds or nuts of your choice

In a blender, place almond milk, protein powder, coconut milk, vanilla, spirulina, maca, and blueberries. Mix liquid with the chia seeds in a container, and allow to sit in the fridge overnight. Stir before serving. Top with berries and mixed nuts.

If you want to change things up, make a simple nut granola. Use sliced almonds, walnuts, cashews, and flax seeds. Coat them in coconut oil, vanilla, and cinnamon and bake in the oven at 325° until crispy, about 10 to 15 minutes.

Asian Fish Salad

Can be made with leftover or canned fish.

Leftover white fish or 2 cans of fish
1 garlic clove, minced
1 teaspoon fresh ginger, powdered or grated
1 juiced lime
2 tablespoons rice vinegar
1 tablespoon toasted sesame oil
1 tablespoon olive oil
1 tablespoon chili paste (or ½ teaspoon chili pepper flakes)
1 tablespoon miso paste (or tahini)
1 cucumber, peeled, sliced longwise and then cut into ¼-inch half moons
1-2 large carrots, shredded
½ red onion, thinly sliced
½ bunch cilantro, chopped
½ bunch scallions, chopped
½ cup cashews, chopped
Salt and pepper to taste

In a large bowl, combine garlic, ginger, lime juice, vinegar, sesame oil, olive oil, chili paste, miso paste, salt and pepper. Mix well.

Stir in the cucumber, carrots, onion, cilantro, scallions, and half the cashews. Then gently mix in the fish without breaking it up to much. Put into a bowl and top with the remaining cashews.

Beanless Chili

For those cold days when you need something filling and heartwarming.

2 yellow onions, thinly sliced

3 bell peppers, thinly sliced

2 carrots, cut lengthwise and then into ½-inch pieces

1 tablespoon paprika

1 tablespoon smoked paprika

1 tablespoon cumin

1 teaspoon chili powder (or more if you like it hot)

1 teaspoon dried oregano

2 lbs. ground beef (or 1 lb. beef and 1 lb. bison)

4 garlic cloves, minced

2 cans diced tomatoes

1 jar tomato sauce

2 cups bone broth or stock

1 bay leaf

1 avocado, sliced

1 bunch cilantro, chopped

Salt and pepper to taste

Saute the onions in a large thick-bottomed pot on medium heat. Once the onions are browned slightly, add in the bell peppers. Add all the spices and the carrots. Stir until the spices become fragrant, about 5 minutes.

Add all the meat and cook until the moisture reduces.

Add in the garlic and cook another 2 minutes. Pour in the diced tomatoes and scrape anything sticking on the bottom of the pan. Add in the tomato sauce and cook for 20 minutes, stirring occasionally.

Pour in the stock and the bay leaf. Cover and reduce the heat to low. Cook for 45 minutes to an hour, stirring every 4 to 5 minutes. Uncover and reduce for 15 more minutes.

Fill the bowls and top with avocado and cilantro.

Beef and Broccoli

Try broccolini or broccoli rabe for a change.

1½ lbs. flank steak, cut into ¼-inch-thick bite-size pieces

1 tablespoon coconut aminos

1 tablespoon rice wine vinegar

4 cups chopped broccoli

2 tablespoons sesame oil

3 garlic cloves, minced

2 tablespoons sesame seeds

½ bunch scallions, chopped

Sauce:

3 tablespoons coconut aminos

1 tablespoon toasted sesame oil

2 teaspoons ginger, minced

2 garlic cloves, minced

1 tablespoon miso paste (or tahini)

2 juiced limes

1-2 tablespoons chili paste or 1 teaspoon chili flakes

Preheat oven to 400°. Mix sauce ingredients together and set aside.

Put the steak in a bowl and add the coconut aminos and vinegar. Allow to marinate for at least 10 minutes, or up to 1 hour.

Put the broccoli in a separate bowl and coat with half of the sauce. Pour the broccoli onto a parchment-lined baking sheet and bake for approximately 30 minutes.

Heat 2 tablespoons of the sesame oil in a large sauté pan on medium-high heat. Once hot, take the meat from the marinade and place in the pan with the garlic. Cook until the meat is browned slightly and is cooked through.

Toss in the cooked broccoli and mix until fully incorporated. Pour in the remaining sauce and the remaining tablespoon of sesame seeds.

Place beef and broccoli on a plate and top with scallions and remaining sesame seeds.

Fried Eggs with Broccoli Beef

Eggs fried over-easy on any leftover protein is my favorite breakfast. Pair Broccoli Beef leftovers with your favorite style of eggs. It's quick, easy, well-balanced, and satisfying.

Balsamic Salad Dressing

Lunch is leftover chili and a salad if you'd like. Here's a balsamic salad dressing you'll love.

¼ cup balsamic vinegar
2 tablespoons Dijon mustard
1 juiced lemon
2 garlic cloves
1 teaspoon fresh or dried thyme
½ cup olive oil
Salt and pepper to taste

Place everything but the olive oil in the blender. Blend until homogenous. Slowly drizzle the oil into the blender while it is running on low. Store in your fridge for up to 2 weeks.

Chicken Thighs with Herbed Cauliflower Rice and Green Sauce

Green Sauce is never the same, and always amazingly delicious. A good sauce can elevate a simple meal to a memorable one, and this one is particularly forgiving and adjustable.

8 bone-in, skin-on chicken thighs (or chicken breasts)

1 tablespoon cumin

1 tablespoon smoked paprika

2 tablespoons salt

1 tablespoon pepper

1 lemon, halved

2 tablespoons ghee or high-heat oil of your choice

1 head cauliflower, grated

2 tablespoons olive oil

3 garlic cloves, minced

¼ cup parsley

¼ cup chives

Green sauce:

Choose 2 different herbs out of the list — there is no wrong combo: scallions, cilantro, parsley, basil, chives, tarragon

1 juiced lemon

3 garlic cloves

¼ cup apple cider vinegar

½ cup olive oil

Salt and pepper to taste

Optional: fresh or dried chili, miso paste instead of salt, ½ peeled apple, orange juice.

Preheat oven to 350°.

Combine the cumin, paprika, salt, and pepper in a bowl and coat the chicken evenly.

In a large sauté pan, heat the ghee on medium high heat. Place as many chicken thighs, skin side down, as will fit comfortably. Once the skin is golden brown, flip the chicken over and brown the other side. If you are doing the chicken in batches, make sure you are not burning the bottom of the pan. If so, wash the pan, and then do the next batch.

Place all the finished chicken skin side up in the pan, tight together. Drizzle with a little more olive oil and set the lemon halves nestled in among the chicken. Put in the oven and cook for 45 minutes to an hour.

While the chicken is cooking, prepare the cauliflower rice and the green sauce.

To make the cauliflower rice, remove the stem and leaves from the cauliflower and discard. Grate the entire head of cauliflower by hand, or place cut pieces of the head in the food processor and process until it is the size of rice grains. Melt coconut oil in a sauté pan over medium heat, add salt and pepper, and stir until heated. For this recipe, add the olive oil and minced garlic at the beginning of the cooking process. At the end, stir in the chives and parsley.

In a blender combine all the green sauce ingredients (use the lemon that has been roasting in the oven with the chicken).

Place cauliflower rice on a plate with the chicken and top it all with a drizzle of green sauce. Keep the sauce in the fridge for up to 5 days.

Savory Cauliflower Porridge with Eggs and Green Sauce

Place the eggs in a pot of water and bring to a boil. Turn off heat and allow to sit in the water for 8 minutes (soft), 10 minutes (medium), or 12 minutes (hard). Make sure to salt the water well.

Heat up the cauliflower rice and place in a bowl topped with the egg and a little green sauce. Mix in a little arugula if you like.

Chicken Salad with Green Goddess Dressing

Leftover chicken (save half for Saturday's dinner)
Salad greens
1 avocado
1 handful cherry tomatoes, halved
¼ cup almonds, toasted and sliced
Leftover green sauce

Debone the leftover chicken from dinner. In a bowl, combine the salad greens, ½ of the avocado, tomatoes, and chicken.

Blend ½ cup green sauce with the other half of the avocado.

Dress the salad (put leftover dressing in the fridge).

Top with toasted almonds.

Ham Hock Pea Soup

It makes the recipe easier if you slow cook the ham hock in stock overnight in a slow cooker.

1 smoked ham hock
2 yellow onions, thinly sliced
3 tablespoons ghee or olive oil
4 parsnips, peeled and cut into ¼-inch half moons
4 garlic cloves, minced
2 teaspoons fresh thyme
1 teaspoon chili pepper flakes
Salt and pepper to taste
2 bags frozen peas, thawed for at least 20 minutes
1 bay leaf
2 containers stock (or 2 quarts homemade)

If you did not slow cook the ham hock overnight, boil the ham in water for an hour to soften.

In a thick-bottomed pot, sauté the onions in ghee or olive oil.

Add in the parsnips, garlic, thyme, pepper flakes, and salt and pepper. Sauté until the garlic is fragrant and the parsnips have softened slightly.

Add in the peas and bay leaf. Stir for 5 minutes, then pour in the stock and add the ham hock.

Cook for 45 minutes on medium-low heat, stirring occasionally.

Remove the ham and use an immersion blender to blend the soup until it is slightly chunky and not quite puréed. If you don't have an immersion blender, pulse the soup in batches in your blender. Be careful not to blend too much.

Shred the ham into small pieces and put the meat back into the soup. Add salt and pepper to taste.

Protein Pancakes

Protein powders are not created equal — read your labels!

1 cup almond flour
¼ cup Whey Clean protein powder
1 cup nut milk or coconut milk
1 egg
2 tablespoons coconut oil, melted (more for cooking)
1 ½ teaspoons baking powder
2 teaspoons vanilla
1 teaspoon cinnamon
Pinch of salt
Berries of your choice

Combine all dry and all wet ingredients in separate bowls. Stir well. Pour the wet ingredients into the dry and stir until just combined.

Heat a cast iron or stainless steel sauté pan on medium heat. Use ghee or coconut oil. Once the oil is hot, scoop dough with a large spoon, making sure there is enough room so that the pancakes don't touch.

Cook until one side is lightly browned, then flip, doing the same on that side.

Top with berries, or blend berries to make syrup.

Chicken Fajitas and Salad

Leftover chicken (or 3 chicken thighs, cooked)

2 tablespoons olive oil

1 red onion, thinly sliced

2 bell peppers, thinly sliced

1 tablespoon cumin

1 tablespoon paprika

1 teaspoon dried oregano

1 teaspoon red pepper flakes

Salt and pepper to taste

4 garlic cloves, minced

2 tablespoons beef fat, duck fat, or other high-heat oil

2 limes

1 bunch cilantro, chopped

1 avocado, sliced

1 jar salsa (optional)

½ bag of salad greens

1 juiced lime

2 garlic cloves, minced

Shred the chicken and set aside.

Heat 2 tablespoons oil in a large sauté pan. Put in the onions and stir for a few minutes. Add in the peppers and all the seasonings and salt and pepper.

Once the peppers and onions are start to soften and turn brown, add the chicken and ½ of the minced garlic to the pan.

When the chicken is hot, and the seasoning is evenly mixed, squeeze in the juice of 1 lime. Turn off the heat and stir in ½ of the chopped cilantro.

In a small bowl, mix the lime juice, remaining garlic, olive oil, and salt and pepper together. Dress your favorite greens lightly.

Set the fajitas onto a plate and top with a slice of lime, cilantro, avocado slices, and a little salsa. Finish with your simple salad and enjoy!

Yam Hash with Fried Eggs

Yams are filled with vitamin C, fiber, potassium, manganese, and metabolic B vitamins.

1 large yam, grated
3 tablespoons ghee
½ yellow onion, thinly sliced
2 garlic cloves, minced
4 eggs
A little of that trusty green sauce or goddess dressing you have leftover
Salt and pepper to taste

Heat 2 tablespoons ghee on medium heat in a large non-stick sauté pan. Add in the onions, and salt them lightly. Once translucent, add in the shredded sweet potato. Stir at first, and then allow to get browned slightly before stirring the mixture again. Once you get a good color on the sweet potato (about 10 to 15 minutes), add in the garlic and a little salt and pepper.

In a separate small non-stick pan, cook your eggs on medium-low heat with the remaining 1 tablespoon of ghee.

Scoop hash onto a plate, top with eggs and a little green sauce if you feel like it.

Kitchen Sink Salad

Kitchen sink salad is exactly how it sounds. Look through your fridge at the end of the week and pull out all the odds and ends you haven't used up. Toss them all together with whatever dressing you want.

If today is your food-shopping day, it is always good to clear out the old stuff before filling your fridge with your groceries for the week.

Kitchen Sink Soup works the same way.

Zucchini Noodles with Bolognese

3 tablespoons olive oil

1 onion, diced

1 carrot, sliced lengthwise and cut into thin half moons

1 stalk celery, finely chopped

½ lb. ground beef

½ lb. ground pork or lamb

4 garlic cloves, minced

1 teaspoon dried oregano

1 teaspoon chili pepper flakes

1 cup red wine 1 can diced tomatoes in their juice

5 zucchini, peeled into long strips like linguine

1 bunch basil

Salt and pepper to taste

Heat a large sauté pan on medium high heat and add the 3 tablespoons olive oil. Once hot, add in the onions. Stir until the onions become translucent, then salt lightly. Add in the carrots and celery. Salt lightly.

Once the carrots are soft, add in the ground meat. Stir until thoroughly cooked and all liquid has evaporated. Add in the garlic, oregano, and chili flakes, and cook until fragrant, about 2 minutes.

Pour in the red wine. Once it is mostly absorbed, pour in the diced tomatoes. Turn the heat to low and simmer for 30 to 45 minutes, stirring occasionally. Salt and pepper to taste.

While the sauce is cooking, peel the zucchini with your peeler, as evenly as you can.

When the sauce is done put half into another pan and stir in the zucchini, stirring them gently into the hot sauce.

Chop basil and top each plate with it.

Keep the zucchini slices and sauce separate if you are eating this meal for lunch the next day. Heat up the sauce and add the noodles right before eating to avoid soggy noodles. Enjoy!

Week 2 Shopping List

Produce:

5 avocadoes

1 head cauliflower

1 large bag carrots

7 lemons

7 limes

7 yellow onions

2 red onions

3 fennel bulbs

7 zucchini

4 parsnips

1 large yam

5 bell peppers

1 bunch celery

2 bunches parsley

2 bunches cilantro

2 bunches scallions

1 bunch chives

1 bunch basil

1 bunch fresh thyme

2 bunches broccoli (or 4 broccolini)

4 parsnips

2 cucumbers

2 heads garlic

1 bulb ginger

1 container cherry tomatoes

2 containers blueberries

1 container blackberries

1 bunch red leaf or bib lettuce

Large bag of your favorite salad greens

1 bag baby kale

1 bag spinach

Canned and bottled goods:

1 can coconut milk

Toasted sesame oil

Ghee

Coconut oil

Beef fat, duck fat, or high-heat oil of your choice

Rice vinegar

Apple cider vinegar

Balsamic vinegar

Coconut aminos (or Bragg's)

3 cans diced tomatoes

1 jar tomato sauce

Dijon mustard

Chili paste (optional)

Meat, eggs, milk:

2 dozen eggs

1 container almond milk (unsweetened)

1 ½ lbs. white sea bass or white fish of your choice

1 smoked ham hock

2 ½ lbs. ground beef

1 ½ lbs. flank steak

½ lb. ground pork or lamb

8 bone-in, skin-on chicken thighs

Dry goods and spices:
Paprika
Smoked paprika
Cumin
Cinnamon
Vanilla
Oregano
Bay leaf
1 bag slivered almonds, raw
1 bag walnuts, raw, halved
1 bag cashews, raw
1 container sesame seeds
1 bag chia seeds
1 bag almond flour
Baking powder
Maca (optional)
Spirulina (optional)

Other:
Brown rice
Miso paste (or tahini)
1 bottle red wine
3 containers stock of your choice
2 bags frozen peas
1 jar salsa (optional)

Week Three

Week 3 Menus

Monday
Breakfast: Veggie and Bacon Omelet
Lunch: Mixed Veggie and Chicken Salad
Dinner: Roman-Style Chicken with Arugula Salad

Tuesday
Breakfast: Eggs with Peppers and Onions
Lunch: Chicken Salad
Dinner: Pan-Seared Salmon with Kale Salad

Wednesday
Breakfast: Nut'ola with Fruit and Coconut Yogurt
Lunch: Salmon and Kale Salad
Dinner: Lamb Meatballs with Sautéed Eggplant and Mint Sauce

Thursday
Breakfast: Eggplant Baked Eggs
Lunch: Lamb Meatballs and Arugula Salad
Dinner: Leek, Mushroom, Chicken and Parsnip Soup

Friday
Breakfast: Nut'ola Smoothie Bowl
Lunch: Leek, Mushroom, Chicken, and Parsnip Soup
Dinner: Turkey Burgers with Sweet Potato Fries

Saturday

Breakfast: Shakshuka

Lunch: Turkey Burgers

Dinner: Beef Curry

Sunday

Breakfast: Crepes

Lunch: Beef Curry

Dinner: Pork Chops with Roasted Apples and Rutabaga Mash

Week 3 Recipes

Veggie and Bacon Omelet

4 eggs
1 tablespoon olive oil
¼ yellow onion, thinly sliced
1 sweet pepper, chopped
1 cup spinach
3 pieces bacon, cooked and broken up
1 tomato, diced
Salt and pepper to taste

Heat a small non-stick pan on medium heat. Add half the olive oil. Sauté the onions and peppers until soft. Salt and pepper.

Whisk the eggs well and pour into the pan with the onions and peppers. Stir gently. Allow edges to set and stir again. Turn heat to low and cover.

Once the eggs are almost set, sprinkle spinach and bacon on top, cover, and turn the heat off.

Once the spinach wilts, fold the omelet over and serve. Top with chopped tomatoes.

Mixed Veggie and Chicken Salad

1 can chicken (or fish)

1-2 large handfuls salad greens

1 avocado, sliced

2 carrots, grated

1 tomato, diced

¼ cup almonds or walnuts, chopped

Salad dressing:

Olive oil, balsamic vinegar, lemon juice, and salt and pepper to taste

Combine all ingredients, mixing lightly. Keep dressing separate until you want to eat, so the greens do not wilt.

Roman-Style Chicken with Arugula Salad

6 bone-in, skin-on chicken thighs

¼ cup olive oil

2 red bell peppers, sliced

2 yellow onions, sliced

3 oz. prosciutto, chopped

4 garlic cloves, minced

1 can diced tomatoes

½ cup white wine

1 tablespoon thyme (fresh is preferred)

1 teaspoon oregano (fresh is preferred)

½ cup chicken stock

2 tablespoons capers

¼ cup parsley, chopped

Salt and pepper to taste

Salad:

2 large handfuls arugula

Top with a little lemon, olive oil, balsamic, salt and pepper

Season the chicken with salt and pepper. In a large sauté pan, heat the olive oil over medium heat. Cook the chicken until brown on both sides. Remove from the pan and set aside.

Add the peppers, onions, and prosciutto into the pan. Cook until the prosciutto is crisp, and the onions and peppers are start to turn brown. Add in the garlic and cook just until fragrant. Add the wine, followed by the tomatoes and herbs. Scrape anything stuck to the bottom of the pan.

Add the chicken back in, and pour in the stock. Cover and cook on low heat for 20 minutes, or until the chicken is cooked all the way through. Top with capers and parsley and serve with arugula salad.

Eggs with Onions and Peppers

4 eggs
1 tablespoon olive oil
Leftover onions and peppers
Salt and pepper to taste
¼ cup parsley, chopped

Heat the olive oil in a non-stick pan over medium heat. Sauté the onions and peppers until hot. Crack the eggs over the mixture without breaking, and salt and pepper it. Cover the pan and cook until the egg whites are cooked and the yolks are still soft, about 4 to 5 minutes.

Use a spatula to scoop mixture onto a plate. Top with parsley.

Chicken Salad

4 chicken thighs, cooked and shredded (2 for now, 2 for soup later in the week)

2-3 large handfuls spinach

1 avocado, sliced

½ cucumber, sliced lengthwise and cut into half moons

¼ cup almonds, sliced

Dressing:

½ juiced lemon

1 tablespoon apple cider vinegar

1 tablespoon olive oil

1 tablespoon whole-grain mustard

Salt and pepper to taste

In a small bowl, combine all dressing ingredients and mix well. In a large bowl, combine all salad ingredients. Mix dressing in if eating immediately, or leave separate until ready to eat.

Pan-Seared Salmon with Kale Salad

This wilted kale salad is great the next day. Kale is sturdy and can stand up to dressings and time. Topped with the cooked salmon, you can enjoy it right away, or put it in a container and bring it to work.

3 salmon filets
2 garlic cloves, minced
2 tablespoons olive oil
½ lemon
Salt and pepper to taste

Kale salad:
¼ cup olive oil
½ yellow onion, sliced
2 bunches kale, chopped, with stems removed
½ juiced lemon
¼ cup walnuts, toasted (spread on baking sheet and heat in a hot oven until they become fragrant – don't burn!)

Add the minced garlic to 1 tablespoon of the olive oil and coat the fish. Salt and pepper both sides. Set aside.

Sauté the onions for the salad in ¼ cup of olive oil. Salt and pepper lightly. Once slightly brown, pour onions and oil over the kale in a heat-resistant bowl, and stir until the kale is fully coated. Add lemon juice and salt and pepper to taste. Set aside.

Heat the remaining 1 tablespoon olive oil in a sauté pan on medium heat. Add the salmon, turning after about 3 minutes. Cook until center is still slightly pink, about 4 more minutes, depending on thickness. Put the salad on a plate, topping with the walnuts. Place the salmon on the plate and squeeze a little bit of the lemon over top.

Nut'ola with Fruit and Coconut Yogurt

Nut'ola can be made in large batches, so it makes future breakfasts quick and easy. I suggest making it on the weekend, while you have time, and keeping it in an airtight glass container. Any nuts can be used — this is not an all-inclusive list. Feel free to add whatever nuts you like and take out something if you don't.

2 cups almonds, sliced
2 cups coconut flakes
1 cup walnuts, chopped
1 cup macadamia nuts
½ cup flax seeds
½ cup chia seeds
½ cup sesame seeds
2 oranges, juiced and zested
¼ cup coconut oil
1 tablespoon vanilla
Salt to taste

Preheat oven to 300°.

Heat the coconut oil, orange juice, zest, cinnamon, and vanilla in a large pot until the zest becomes fragrant. Add in all the nuts, seeds, and coconut flakes, stirring until coated. Salt lightly.

Line 2 sheet trays with parchment and spread the mixture over the 2 trays. Cook until browned slightly, stirring every 10 minutes so it doesn't burn on the edges.

Allow to cool completely before putting into an airtight container.

To serve, place coconut yogurt in a bowl, sprinkle the Nut'ola over the yogurt, and then top with your favorite berries.

For more protein, mix Whey Clean protein powder into your yogurt before you top with nuts and berries.

Lamb Meatballs with Sautéed Eggplant and Mint Sauce

2 lbs. ground lamb

4 garlic cloves, minced

1 tablespoon cumin

1 teaspoon paprika

1 teaspoon smoked paprika

¼ teaspoon cayenne

1 ½ teaspoons salt

1 teaspoon pepper

1 egg

Eggplant:

3 eggplants, diced large

4 tablespoons olive oil

3 garlic cloves, minced

Salt and pepper to taste

Mint sauce:

2 bunches mint

2 garlic cloves

1 juiced lemon

3 tablespoons apple cider vinegar

¼ cup olive oil

Salt and pepper to taste, add cayenne if you want it to be spicy

Preheat oven to 350°.

Salt the eggplant and allow it to sit in a colander to get rid of excess moisture. Dab with a paper towel periodically.

Combine the lamb, garlic, all the spices, salt, pepper, and the egg. Mix until fully combined. Roll into golf-ball-size meatballs.

Heat a large cast iron pan on medium-high heat. Add 2 tablespoons olive oil to the pan and allow to heat up. Add all the meatballs to the pan — it's ok if they're snug. Allow to brown. Using tongs, flip meatballs over. Put the meatballs in the oven to finish cooking, about 20 minutes.

Heat the 4 tablespoons olive oil in a large sauté pan on medium heat. Add the eggplant and sauté until browned and softened, about 15 to 20 minutes. Add in the garlic, salt, and pepper, and sauté until fragrant.

Blend the mint sauce ingredients in a blender until smooth.

Remove the meatballs from the oven. Put the eggplant on a plate with the meatballs, and top with mint sauce.

Eggplant Baked Eggs

4 eggs
Leftover eggplant
2 tablespoons olive oil
Salt and pepper to taste
¼ cup parsley

Heat a non-stick pan over medium heat and add the olive oil. Add the eggplant and stir until hot. Crack the eggs over the eggplant, keeping the yolks intact. Salt and pepper lightly, then cover, turning to low heat.

Cook until whites are solid and yolk is still soft. Top with parsley and serve.

Leek, Mushroom, Chicken, and Parsnip Soup

2 chicken thighs, cooked and shredded

3 tablespoons olive oil

1 yellow onion, sliced

4 parsnips, peeled, sliced lengthwise, and cut into half moons

3 leeks, green tops removed, white parts sliced

8-12 cremini mushrooms, thinly sliced

3 garlic cloves, minced

1 teaspoon thyme (fresh if possible)

1 container chicken or vegetable stock

½ juiced lemon

½ cup parsley, chopped

Salt and pepper to taste

Heat a thick-bottomed pot over medium-high heat. Add the olive oil. Sauté the onions until translucent, salting lightly. Add the parsnips and leeks. Cook until the parsnips are softened slightly, about 5 minutes. Add in the mushrooms, salting lightly. Add the garlic and thyme, cooking until fragrant.

Pour in the chicken stock and turn the heat down to medium low, cooking slowly until parsnips are soft. About 20 to 30 minutes. Add in the cooked and shredded chicken. Add in the lemon juice and the parsley. Enjoy.

Nut'Ola Smoothie Bowl

½ cup nut'ola

½ cup frozen berries

¼ cup unsweetened almond or coconut milk

1 cup spinach

¼ cup Whey Clean protein powder

1 teaspoon spirulina (optional)

1 tablespoon maca (optional)

Place berries, coconut milk, spinach, protein powder, spirulina and maca in the blender. Blend until smooth. Put in a bowl and top with nut'ola.

Turkey Burgers with Sweet Potato Fries

2 lbs. ground turkey, portioned into patties

Mustard

2 tomatoes, sliced

½ red onion, thinly sliced

1 head bib lettuce, separated carefully for lettuce wraps

2 sweet potatoes, peeled, cut in half and sliced into ¼-inch strips

¼ cup olive oil

2 garlic cloves, minced

Salt and pepper to taste

Preheat oven to 400°.

Toss the sweet potato fries in enough olive oil to coat, along with the minced garlic, salt, and pepper. Spread onto a parchment-lined baking sheet, and bake, stirring halfway through cooking. Allow to brown lightly but not to burn, about 20 minutes.

Meanwhile, heat the remaining olive oil in a large cast iron pan on medium-high heat. Generously salt and pepper the turkey burger patties. Cook the patties until nicely browned on both sides. Put in the oven for 10 minutes to cook through.

Put a patty in a lettuce leaf, top with mustard, tomato, and sliced onion, and enjoy with the crispy sweet potato fries.

Shakshuka

Shakshuka is an Israeli dish that is immensely flavorful, simple, and colorful. It also makes a great quick dinner over a bed of arugula or kale.

4 eggs
2 tablespoon olive oil
1 yellow onion, sliced
2 red bell peppers, sliced
1 teaspoon smoked paprika
1 teaspoon cumin
Salt, pepper, and cayenne to taste
4 garlic cloves, minced
3 tomatoes, diced
Leftover sweet potato (optional)
1 bunch parsley, chopped
1 tablespoon paprika

Heat oven to 350°.

Heat olive oil in a cast iron pan over medium-high heat. Sauté the onions and peppers until softened. Add in the paprika, smoked paprika, cumin, salt, and pepper, stirring until fragrant. Add in the garlic and cook for 2 minutes. Add the tomatoes and optional potatoes, scraping the bottom to loosen anything stuck to the pan.

Crack the eggs onto the mixture, keeping the yolks intact. Salt and pepper lightly. Place in the oven for 10 minutes, or until the eggs reach your desired doneness. Top with parsley and serve.

Turkey Burger with Spinach Salad

Bib lettuce, ripped into bite-size pieces
1-2 large handfuls spinach
1 tomato, diced
½ cucumber, sliced into ¼-inch half moons
Leftover turkey burger patties
1 tablespoon olive oil

Dressing:
2 tablespoons Dijon mustard
2 tablespoons apple cider vinegar
½ juiced lemon
1 garlic clove, minced
3 tablespoons olive oil
Salt and pepper to taste

Put the bib lettuce, spinach, tomatoes, and cucumber in a bowl. In a separate small bowl, whisk the dressing ingredients together.

Heat a sauté pan on medium heat. Add the olive oil and cook the leftover turkey burger patties until warm through, about 4 minutes on each side.

Dress the salad, saving a little for the burger. Place the salad on a plate and top with the turkey burger, drizzling the remaining dressing over the burger.

Beef Curry

Curry is one of those dishes that's even better the next day, so make extra!

2 lbs. beef chuck or tri-tip, cut into 1-inch pieces

4 tablespoons ghee

3 yellow onions, diced

3 tablespoons curry powder

1 tablespoon cumin

1 tablespoon coriander

1 tablespoon cinnamon

1 apple, peeled and grated

2 tablespoons ginger, grated

6 garlic cloves, minced

1 juiced lemon

1 container chicken stock

3 large carrots, peeled, cut into inch-thick circles

1 kabocha squash, peeled, seeded, and chopped into 1-inch pieces

Salt and pepper to taste

Fresh chopped cilantro

Generously salt and pepper the beef chunks. Heat a large heavy-bottomed pot on medium-high heat. Add the ghee and allow it to get hot. Brown the meat, working in batches. Do not crowd the pan, or the meat will not get the proper sear, which gives you that rich, full flavor. Brown well on all sides, then set the batch aside until all the beef is done.

Leaving the beef aside, sauté the onions in the hot pot. Once the onions are translucent, add in all the spices and salt and pepper. Add the apple, scraping the bottom of the pot with a wooden spoon to stop the mixture from burning. Add in the ginger, garlic, and lemon juice, stirring well.

Add the beef and pour the stock into the pot. Simmer until the beef is almost tender (approximately 45 minutes) then add in the carrots and squash.

Cook for another 30-45 minutes, or until the carrots and squash are tender and the beef is juicy. Taste and adjust seasoning if necessary. Serve with fresh chopped cilantro.

Crepes

4 scoops Whey Clean protein powder

6 egg whites

½ zested lemon

1 tsp vanilla

Salt to taste

Coconut oil or ghee for the pan

Toppings:

Coconut yogurt

Berries

Whisk the egg whites with the lemon zest, vanilla, and salt. Once small bubbles start to form, whisk in the protein powder.

Heat a non-stick pan, lightly coated with coconut oil or ghee, on medium heat.

Pour a small ladle of batter into the pan. Lift the pan and tilt it, spreading the batter evenly to all the edges. Cook for 2 to 3 minutes or until just cooked. Using a spatula, flip the crepe, and cook through, about 3 more minutes.

Fill the crepes with yogurt and berries. If you want to make a sauce, heat the berries up until softened.

Pork Chop with Roasted Apples and Rutabaga Mash

Rutabaga is a cross between a cabbage and a turnip. Perhaps the most important function of rutabagas involves their diverse composition of antioxidant compounds, notably glucosinolates, which are somewhat rare sulfur-containing compounds that have been shown to reduce the growth of cancerous tumors in the body. Furthermore, their high levels of carotenoids and vitamin C act as antioxidants, which combat the effects of free radicals, thereby preventing the mutation of healthy cells into cancerous cells, among other effects. Rutabagas can effectively prevent premature aging, improve eyesight, and stimulate the healthy regeneration of cells throughout our organs and tissues.

2 pork chops

3 rutabagas, peeled and cut into 1/2-inch-thick pieces

1 yellow onion, thinly sliced

4 garlic cloves, minced

4 tablespoons olive oil

2 tablespoons fresh thyme

2 apples, peeled and thinly sliced

1 juiced lemon

Handful of parsley, chopped

Salt and pepper to taste

Preheat oven to 350°. Salt and pepper the pork chops and set aside.

Toss the rutabagas and ½ of the onions in a bowl with ½ of the minced garlic cloves and ½ of the olive oil. Salt and pepper generously. Pour onto a parchment-lined baking sheet and roast until the rutabagas are tender, approximately 45 minutes.

Meanwhile, heat a cast iron pan on medium-high heat using the remaining olive oil or ghee. Sear the pork chop until golden brown on both sides. Sprinkle ½ of the thyme over the pork chops and place in the oven for 15 minutes, or until center is just slightly pink.

Remove the pork chops from the pan, and grill the remaining onions in the pan over medium heat. Once the onions are translucent, add the apples, ½ of the remaining garlic, lemon juice, and the remaining thyme. Salt and pepper lightly.

Place the rutabaga mixture, ½ of the parsley, and the remaining garlic into a food processor and pulse until smooth.

Slice the pork chop against the grain and serve on a plate with the mash. Top with the grilled apples and a sprinkle of parsley.

Week 3 Shopping List

Produce:

1 large bunch spinach

1 large bunch arugula

4 bunches kale

1 head bib lettuce

4 bunches parsley

2 bunches mint

1 bunch cilantro

1 bunch fresh thyme

8 lemons

4 oranges

2 heads garlic

1 large piece ginger

9 yellow onions

1 red onion

3 large leeks

3-4 avocadoes

6-7 large carrots

4 red bell peppers

2 large sweet potatoes

4 large parsnips

3 large rutabagas

1 kabocha squash

8-12 cremini mushrooms (depending on size)

3 large eggplants

3 apples

1 large cucumber

8 tomatoes

2 containers blueberries

2 containers blackberries

2 containers raspberries

Canned and bottled goods:

1 jar whole grain mustard

1 jar Dijon mustard

1 bottle apple cider vinegar

1 bottle balsamic vinegar

1 bottle olive oil

1 jar coconut oil

1 jar ghee

1 jar capers

1 can diced tomatoes

1 can chicken (or fish)

3 containers chicken stock

Meat, eggs, milk:

2 dozen eggs

1 qt. almond milk, cashew milk, or coconut milk

1 large container unsweetened coconut or almond milk Yogurt

1 pkg. bacon

2 pork chops

10 bone-in, skin-on chicken thighs

2 lbs. ground lamb

2 lbs. ground turkey

2 lbs. beef chuck or tri-tip

3 salmon filets

¼ lb. prosciutto

Dry goods and spices:

Vanilla

1 bag sliced almonds

1 bag halved walnuts

1 bag large coconut flakes

1 bag flax seeds

1 bag chia seeds

1 jar sesame seeds

1 jar cumin

1 jar paprika

1 jar smoked paprika

1 jar coriander

1 jar cayenne

1 jar oregano

1 jar curry powder

1 large jar cinnamon

1 small container maca powder (optional)

1 small container spirulina powder (optional)

Other:

Whey Clean Protein Powder (available at www.CleanKUT.com)

1 bottle white wine

1 bag mixed frozen berries

Getting Started

You are what you do, not what you say you'll do.
-C.G. Jung

Are you overwhelmed yet? I know there's a lot of information here, but don't let your fear of the unknown stop you from taking action. Just follow these simple instructions:

1. Print out the Clean Food Levels, and choose which one you will do for 21 days.

2. Make a commitment and write it down. Take time to identify your Big Why.

3. Tell a friend or better yet, enlist an accountability partner.

4. Clean out your kitchen of all foods not on your Clean Food List.

5. Block off time in your calendar this week for shopping, preparing, cooking, and eating. Yes, write it in! You are worth it.

6. Choose a menu plan for your first week by creating your own or using the one provided.

7. Make a shopping list and go get it!

8. Prepare what you can in advance to make meal-time prep easier during the week.

9. Make some food and enjoy!

Mastery Tips

- Focus on what you *can* eat

- Get support, enroll a friend or family member

- When you want a snack, drink a glass of water first

- Make your own salad dressing

Salad Dressing

People love dressing and there aren't many commercial dressings out there that are good. Read your labels and be horrified.

What is a good recipe for salad dressing? Well, here is more of a formula than a recipe:

$$Fat + Acid = Yumminess$$

A good fat choice is any of the oils found on the Clean Food List, such as avocado oil, walnut oil, olive oil, etc. The flavor of your oil will determine the taste of your dressing. If you have not made dressing before, I suggest you start with a good quality Extra Virgin Olive (EVO) oil.

Use your nose. If you don't like the smell of the oil, you are not going to like the taste of it! Oh, and oils go rancid. So if you have oils in your cupboard that have been there for a long time, and they don't smell great, get rid of them.

Once you have chosen your oil, add your favorite acid. An acid is any type of vinegar or fresh citrus juice like lemon (my personal favorite). Again, the flavor of your dressing is determined by what you choose, so be creative until you find something you love.

How much fat and how much acid? The amounts of both are completely up to you. Taste as you go. If it's too tart, add more oil. Too greasy? Add more acid. Whisk, shake, or blend with salt and pepper, and you will never want to buy commercially-made salad dressing again. Really.

For a little variety in your vinaigrette, add garlic and/or Dijon mustard, or a couple of raspberries. Want a creamy dressing? Add avocado and use your blender.

Have fun and enjoy!

Troubleshooting

*Truth is ever to be found in simplicity, and not in the multiplicity
and confusion of things.*
- Isaac Newton

Okay, so you can eat clean when you make your own food, but what happens if you want to eat out or attend a special event? Here are some answers to the most frequently asked questions that I get, along with some simple strategies to support your success.

How do I eat clean at a restaurant?

I love to eat at home rather than a restaurant whenever I can, since I prefer grass-fed, organic, pastured, sustainable, and humanely raised animal products. That being said, it's nice to go out sometimes, right?

It's easy to eat clean in a restaurant if you ask enough questions. Don't be afraid to ask how a dish is prepared. First of all, look for veggies and proteins with the simplest preparations like a salad with grilled fish for example. Words like grilled or steamed tend to be cleaner than fried or sautéed. On most menus you will find a salad or side of veggies that you can add your favorite protein to, so keep it simple and avoid sauces that use mystery oils and sugars.

Many restaurants add oil products to their food to finish them off — it makes them look better and taste juicier. Just ask for it plain.

Personally, I think that everyone should work in a restaurant at some point in their lives so they can see the industrial oils and processed items that restaurants use behind the scene. Restaurants can't make everything from scratch. They are in business to make money, and they have many things to consider when designing their menus, including the cost and availability of ingredients, as well as storage, delivery, and labor. Your health is not necessarily a priority in the mix.

I was getting some Indian food from the hot deli case at my local "health food" grocery store, and I asked if it was gluten-free. The person helping me did not say, "Let me ask the chef," she said, "Oh, let me go read the package." True story.

What do I do on special occasions?

What do you do when you want to eat clean, and you are invited to a party or someone's house for dinner? Of course you can eat before so you are not hungry when you arrive, or better yet, take something with you. I offer to bring a dish that just so happens to be something that I am excited to eat as well.

Not drinking alcohol at a party used to be a little trickier, as I didn't want to call attention to myself about it. I would make a point of sipping on a glass of sparkling water on ice with a wedge and umbrella, until I realized nobody really cared what I was drinking or not drinking. Ha!

What if I live with others who don't eat clean?

I get asked a lot about how to eat clean when you live with family members or roommates who eat differently. This is challenging to be sure, but not impossible. First of all, ask for support from any adults you live with by sharing what you are doing and your Big Why. Then negotiate with them to keep away any of their foods that you might find tempting or difficult to be around.

If you live with kids, start serving more clean meals and let all that pretend food disappear on its own. It has been my experience that if you make a big deal about it, it's a big deal. If you don't, it's not. And they will learn to love real food too.

How do I lose weight?

When you say that you want to lose weight, I am assuming it's excess body fat that you want to lose, right? Because weight loss is easy if you stop eating — but that is extremely unhealthy, as you lose muscle and bone density, and you'll stress vital organ tissue before you hit body fat.

A couple of keys to fat loss:

#1 - You need to eat!! If you restrict calories, your body will think it is starving and will desperately hang on to your body fat, because it wants to survive. Think about it. If you were stranded on an island with nothing to eat, your body would have to live on whatever body fat you have on you right now.

The heavier you are, the more days you have. Great. Except you're not on a desert island.

#2 - Eat CLEAN. Processed, pretend foods provide calories but are not nutrient-dense like real food. To eat clean, you must eat food that your body recognizes as real. Interestingly, research has shown that most people struggling with extra body fat are actually malnourished — overfed but undernourished. They're eating a lot of empty calories that don't have much nutrition. That is why we have so many food cravings. Our stomachs tell us that we're full, but our brain tells us we still need to eat, because we're missing important nutrients.

Bottom line? Eat clean. Move. Sleep. Eat some more. Have fun. Repeat.

How do I know if I'm eating too much or too little?

This question gets asked a lot, because many people have lost touch with their bodies and don't really know how they feel, or should feel. I get asked, "What is a normal portion size?" or "How much should I eat?"

As we clean up our diet and get healthier, we start to have a greater sense of what we want and need. We get to experience self-mastery and begin to trust our own body wisdom to let us know what is best for us. Perhaps your body needs some Vitamin K, so you begin to crave Brussels sprouts. Cool, right?

Until then, out-of-whack hormones can be telling us all kinds of things that may not be supportive. Yes, your brain might be telling you that you need another plate of nachos for dinner, but that is most definitely not the best choice. So when do we get to trust the difference?

Trust your clean food cravings. Also, to balance out your hormone signaling, eat clean meals at regular times throughout your day. Let your body trust you first by feeding it what it needs.

Regardless of which level you're doing on the Clean Food Diet, make sure you're getting the nutrition you need through real food. To begin, you will want to eat a minimum of 3 servings of protein a day (4 to 8 oz. each). The amount really depends on how hungry you are. At each meal, eat at least 1 tablespoon of fat and 1 to 3 cups of veggies.

What if I'm not hungry? Can I skip a meal?

When you have developed a certain degree of body wisdom, I think it is totally fine to skip meals here and there. This is called intermittent fasting, and there are actually some great benefits to it.

However, a lot of people don't feel hungry because they have sluggish digestion and a slow metabolism, which are the very reasons why they should eat. Eating clean food every 4 to 5 hours helps to regulate digestion and speeds up metabolism.

At the beginning of your Clean Food Diet journey, decide on an eating schedule and stick to it. It is a great day when you notice that you are physically hungry. That means things are moving!

If you get hungry between meals, have a snack. Eventually, you will find the eating rhythm that works best for you.

Remember, you don't need to worry about weighing and measuring your food. Go for protein about the size of your palm, fat the size of your thumb, and as many handfuls of veggies as you can eat. Using that as a guideline and making adjustments according to your hunger level will help you cultivate your own body wisdom.

How is this different from an elimination diet?

The Clean Food Diet is a type of elimination diet, cutting out many known inflammatory foods. However, there are other foods that could also be causing distress for certain people who suffer, for instance, with autoimmune disease. Some of these other problematic foods can be:

- Nightshades: tomatoes, eggplant, white potatoes, peppers, and peppery spices.
- Eggs
- Pork

The bottom line is that if you are ill, see a physician. Keep a detailed record of everything you eat and how you feel before and after each meal. You may notice that you feel better when you eliminate these troublesome foods.

How do I know if I am getting enough fiber?

I know that this is a cover question for, "How do I make sure I have a regular bowel movement?" Good. Finally, we are getting to my favorite subject: digestion and elimination. Just ask my students, I love to talk about poop.

First of all, let me tell you that if you are not having at least one significant bowel movement every single day, you need help. A healthy body eliminates waste every day. If you don't, there is something wrong. No one wants to talk about it, but of course I will.

Fiber does not make your bowels move. Fiber is *what* your bowels move. Peristalsis is the name for the muscular contractions that move food throughout your entire digestive system from your esophagus and stomach through your small intestine and colon. These wave-like movements are impacted by the types of foods we eat, the amount of food we eat, and the frequency of which we eat them.

The key is to get dietary fiber from the foods that will support healthy peristalsis and not cause too much distress in the process. Fiber is an important part of the Clean Food Diet and comes from eating whole fruits and veggies.

Most of us were taught that the best dietary fiber comes from grains, and although whole grains do have a lot of fiber, they also have a lot of anti-nutrients and cause irritation to the lining of the gut. Sorry, they do more harm than good.

So eat your greens, drink lots of water, and grab a handful of berries for good measure. You will get all the fiber you need.

If you are still having issues with constipation, there may be some damage from years of unhealthy food choices that need to be looked at. I am here to tell you that it doesn't have to remain this way! Your body can recover. Get the help you need and get moving. Literally.

After 21 Days

The chains of habit are too weak to be felt until they are too strong to be broken.
- Samuel Johnson

Congratulations. After 21 days of cleaner eating, regardless of what level you played at, you are now a healthier version of yourself.

So now what? First of all, take some time to reflect on what you have accomplished and write down your experience. This is important because you will forget, I promise you. Ask a mother who has given birth a second time. Lying there on the delivery table for round two, I thought to myself, "Am I an idiot? This really hurts!" If we can forget something as momentous as the pain of childbirth, we can certainly forget the challenges and victories of altering our food choices for three weeks.

What has changed for you? What was easier than you thought it would be? What was difficult? What results can you see? What results can you not see but you can feel?

Taking time to be mindful will train your brain to collect the positive evidence you need to continue on your clean eating journey.

Yes. Continue.

Remember at the beginning of this book we talked about habitual nourishment? You've laid a great foundation of new habits. Now it's time to build on that.

The good news is, the hardest part is over. The first few weeks of eating clean and reducing the sugar that your body was addicted to is the most challenging. And you did it. Now it's time for another decision. My recommendation is to make another 21-day commitment and choose what Clean Food Diet level you would like to play at this time.

If you started at Beginner or 80/20, and you still have some more body fat you want to lose, or inflammation you want to bring down, then perhaps you are ready to "level up" to Clean KUT? It's your choice. Again, you need to set yourself up for success, so it's just fine to do another three weeks at your current level.

The benefit of doing Clean KUT is that by eliminating foods that are known to cause inflammation, you could actually be healing something inside you that you were not aware of. For instance, let's say that you follow Clean KUT and eliminate dairy for 21 days and are feeling great. Then you eat some ice cream and notice your sinuses are stuffing up a little bit. You are having a reaction to the dairy that you didn't notice before when your diet was not as clean. This is a good thing, because it informs your innate body wisdom.

Maintenance

What if you've reached your goals, or arrived at your ideal body weight, and you feel like a million bucks? Keep on keeping on, my friend. It's time to maintain your amazing results.

You can keep eating at the Clean KUT level for the rest of your life, but I have found that 80/20 is where most people like to hang out. It's the level where you are eating clean most of the time, with the occasional this or that.

"It's not what you do some of the time that counts; it's what you do all of the time that counts." – Jack LaLanne

For me, life is better with dark chocolate, so my Clean Food Diet includes it occasionally. The healthy body knows how to handle a little extra sugar or processed food once in a while. The same holds true if you were to accidently eat a cardboard box — your body would deal with it as best it could. We just want to avoid the compound effects of eating inflammatory foods repeatedly over a period of time.

That being said, BEWARE: slippery slope ahead.

If you still look at a plate of brownies with love in your eyes and consider them to be a real "treat," you must use great caution before you start including them in your diet.

Things to watch for:

1. Over Confidence. If you haven't written out your journey, you may have forgotten what it took to get to this place, and it will seem like nothing. This selective memory often seduces people into, what I call the "I'll Just Clean It Up Again Later" syndrome.

    Eating sugar (simple carbs) triggers the hormones in your brain that make you want to eat more. All the best intentions in the world will not necessarily stop the cascade of impulses that pull you off the road and into the nearest drive-thru.

2. Boredom. If you're bored with what you are eating, consider this. It's not your diet that's boring, you are. The Clean Food Diet has such a variety of foods that there are literally hundreds of thousands of meal

preparations and combinations that are full of flavor and culinary excitement for those interested in trying something new.

Look for recipes, try some ethnic foods, make an effort! The clean food pool is huge and is waiting for you to dive in.

3. Lack of Focus. Perhaps you started feeling better and forgot you ever felt bad, so you take your eye off the meatball. That's understandable. It just means that it's time to revisit your Big Why. If you go back to eating the way you were, you will end up where you've already been. And just to remind you, you didn't like it there.

    What if you know your Big Why, but you start feeling a little lazy and want to grab a box of something and stick it in the microwave anyway? It's time to make it Bigger.

Reintroducing Foods

On the Clean KUT list, we cut out several foods that you may want to eat again: dairy, legumes, and grains. Let's review each one so you can decide if it's a good idea.

When trying to eat foods that are not a part of your Clean Food Diet, it would serve you well to take your time. Introduce only one food at a time so you can notice how it is affecting you physically, mentally, and emotionally.

Dairy

Dairy intolerance can be a problem with digesting either lactose or casein. Studies confirm that 75% of the world's population loses the enzymes needed to break down lactose, and they may not even know it. This translates into severe or mild symptoms, such as skin problems, headaches, asthma, irritable bowel, bloating, gas, persistent cough, colds, and flu.

Sure, you might be one of the lucky 25% that has the mutated gene that can tolerate lactose, but then again, you might not.

To make matters worse, modern farming practices include pasteurization, which kills bacteria, making dairy more stable and longer lasting. But it also kills the enzymes that help make it digestible.

With this in mind, if you are committed to reintroducing dairy into your diet, try to get your hands on whole, raw products from healthy, grass-fed animals. Avoid reduced fat content and pasteurization. Raw milk products are illegal in some states, but do your homework on this. Some people have formed co-ops to find ways around these laws.

Another form of dairy that is easier to tolerate is fermented dairy, such as raw milk yogurt, kefir, and cultured buttermilk.

Nowadays, there are many alternatives to dairy that are easy to fall in love with: coconut milk/cream and almond milk, for example.

Legumes

Legumes are very difficult to digest, and although there are proven traditional preparations that make them absorb easier, the process is time consuming. The phytic acid and enzyme inhibitors in legumes require them to be soaked for 12 to 24 hours and then cooked for another 4 to 8 hours.

Sprouting and fermenting are other ways to work with legumes. If you are missing your beans, then take the time to prepare them properly and have a small portion. Just don't forget to track how you feel afterwards.

Grains

Bread, pasta, pastries, and cereal . . . Miss any of those? They tend to be the most challenging for people to avoid, and those are just the wheat products. Grains include corn and rice products as well.

Before the advent of commercial yeast and processed grains, traditional cultures soaked, sprouted, and fermented grains in order to make them usable. Industrial kitchens that use these techniques are difficult to find, as is learning how to do them yourself, but it is not impossible if you are super committed. Are you?

If you are going to reintroduce grains, I recommend permanently staying away from gluten products, which contain an additional difficult-to-digest plant protein.

Probably the most benign grain product is white rice, because its anti-nutrients and gut irritants have been stripped away. However, it means that white rice does not have any fiber or micronutrients, either.

So, although white rice may be a good way to get some extra calories when you need them, they should not displace other nutrient-dense foods.

The traditional preparation of legumes and grains is a fascinating and delicious art form that I myself have not dedicated the time to master. If it is important to you, do your research, put on your apron, and enjoy!

Your New Normal

The only way to keep your positive results and build upon them is to adopt the Clean Food Diet as part of your lifestyle. This is a mindset that often takes a mind shift in order to happen.

Mindset Mastery Tips:

- Keep your Big Why current and juicy.
- Strengthen your beliefs by continuing to educate yourself. For instance, if you don't believe that grains are impossible to digest and that they wreak havoc on your system, you will eventually justify eating them. Do the research, and get the data you need to solidify your new lifestyle.
- Practice mindfulness every day.
- Surround yourself with healthy, positive people.

- Become someone's mentor and encourage them along their Clean Food Diet journey. Yes, you can.

The Real Deal

Nullum Gratuitum Prandium.
- Latin for "No Free Lunch"

There's a big price tag attached to the Clean Food Diet. I'm not talking about the price of this book. Buying clean food such as organic and grass-fed products can be more expensive than conventional and factory-made pretend food, but that is still not the big price I am referring to. Eating in accordance to the Clean Food Diet will cost you more than money. It will cost you time, energy, self-control, and maybe a few of your precious deep-fried corn dogs and slushy drinks along the way.

There is also a big price to pay if you do not do the Clean Food Diet. Ultimately, it could cost you your life.

Oh, that sounds so dramatic . . . but we are all going to die, right? Some people tell me that life would not be worth living if they couldn't eat what they want (which is almost always some kind of junk food). Wow. That's like a smoker knowing that smoking will kill him or her, but preferring to die rather than live without cigarettes.

Yes, we are all going to die. The balancing act becomes how to enjoy the moment and yet still plan for the future. That is what the Clean Food Diet is — an investment in your future. Sure there are the short term, feel good benefits like fitting into your skinny jeans, but I'm talking about wellness and longevity.

The way I look at it, I can spend time in the kitchen preparing clean food, or spend time in the waiting room at my doctor's office. I can miss out on that easy premade frozen lasagna dinner, or miss out on hiking Yosemite with my grandkids.

It's a choice. What price are you willing to pay? There's no free lunch.

Eating gives us all pleasure and that's awesome. But here's the rub. If eating dinner is the most exciting part of your day, then it's time to get a life. It's time for an inventory of what you want and why you're here. It's time to find your true passion(s) in life.

Food is a sorry substitute for a juicy and fulfilling life. And on top of that, worrying about your weight and obsessing about your body is another distraction that is keeping you from living your big life.

Unclear about your higher purpose? That's okay, but it does not take away your responsibility for it. The opportunity here is to give up those old limiting beliefs that keep you stuck, and to step forward into who you really are.

One of those limiting beliefs is your need for perfection. You are not perfect. You will never be perfect. The expectation to look perfect and eat perfect is just an easy excuse to give up on your Clean Food Diet lifestyle or not do it all. The truth is, you actually are perfect in all your imperfection, and making peace with that is the greatest gift you can give yourself.

Another limiting belief that can keep you stuck is the notion that your problems are all about food. Yes, having a healthy body is foundational (we talked about this at the beginning of the book), but there are lots of things that you are hungry for that are not related to food.

Feed Yourself PIES

The key to creating your dream body and living the life you've always wanted is getting the nourishment you need in every area of your life: Physically, Intellectually, Emotionally, and Spiritually. There are more ways to feed yourself than through your pie hole.

MASTER MEL'S PIES CHART

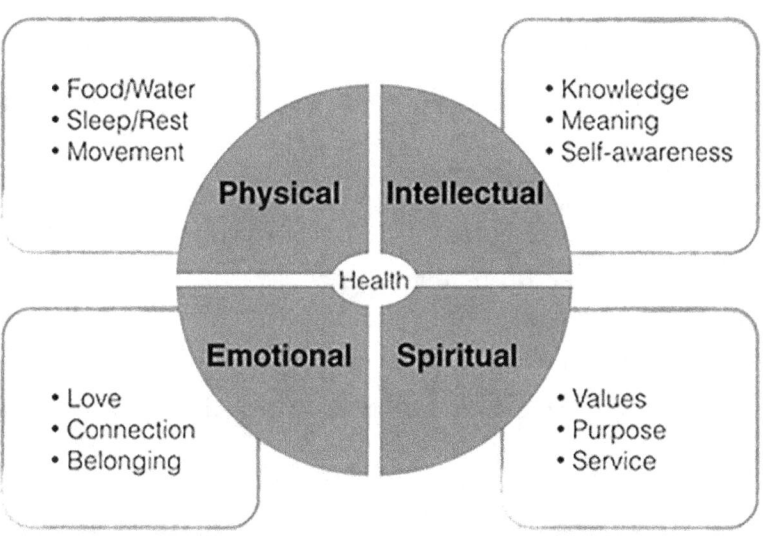

If you are hungry for love and connection, it makes no sense to feed yourself popcorn and pizza. Yet we do it all the time. That's okay.

Emotional hunger requires emotional nutrition and we get that through healthy and loving relationships with friends and family; we get that with a sense of belonging and connectedness with others. If you are not getting the emotional nutrition that you need, or worse, you are not even aware of your emotional needs, it can lead to thoughts and behaviors that reduce your freedom and capacity to experience love.

The same goes for our innate hunger for learning and meaning in life. We must attend to these urges and feed ourselves with knowledge that will fuel our intellect and nurture our mind. Pretzels don't do it.

What is spiritual hunger? Have you ever had an ache or emptiness inside, wondering what this life is really all about? That's the hunger for purpose. It's the desire to be a part of something greater than ourselves — something of value. You know deep down you are here to make a difference and be of service in some significant way. It's time to feed your soul.

Self-mastery is all about learning about yourself — learning about what you need in every area of your life, and finding the way to meet those needs for the benefit of all.

Self-mastery is a lifelong journey. Continue to feed yourself PIES and enjoy your big, juicy, purpose-filled life!

Join me, and other students of self-mastery — let's work together to build a better body, a better life and a better world. Check it out at www.MasterMel. com/CFD

BONUS CHAPTER:

Myth Busting 101

People learn something every day, and a lot of times it's what they
learned the day before was wrong.
- Bill Vaughan

There are so many misconceptions about nutrition. Essentially, we learned a bunch of misinformation through the years that we never bothered to question. I want to share some of my favorite nutritional myths and bring you up to date.

Myth #1: "Eating fat makes you fat."

It's time to put this myth to rest once and for all. Fat is an important part of a healthy diet. In fact, eating healthy fat keeps us healthy. The composition of our brain is 60% fat, and although we absolutely need fats for our brain to function properly, our bodies cannot produce them. We must get these essential fatty acids (EFAs) from what we eat.

Fat also helps us absorb important vitamins and nutrients, and they are essential to our nervous system. The monounsaturated fats in olives, olive oils, and avocados help prevent belly fat, and help protect our arteries from the buildup of plaque. The polyunsaturated fats found in fish and seeds help boost our immune system. The omega-3 fatty acids in grass-fed meat help to normalize thyroid function, increase our metabolic rate, increase muscle mass, and decrease body fat. Fats also play a crucial role in reducing inflammation, protecting against viruses and bacteria, and helping the absorption of micronutrients.

The list of fat benefits goes on and on. As an added bonus, healthy fats keep our appetites satisfied longer, so we don't overindulge. Have you ever noticed you can keep reaching for another basket of bread at a restaurant, but when you have a small cut of steak, you actually feel satisfied? Well, healthy fats keep us feeling full far longer than refined carbohydrates and other junk. Don't shy away from foods in the Clean Food Diet just because of the fat content — your body needs that fat.

It is true that fat has more calories than carbs or proteins, but keep in mind, the foods you see at the store labeled "fat-free" are loaded with sugar and chemicals, which are the real culprits. Eating fat doesn't make you fat. Instead, start looking at fat as something that is satisfying, nutritious, and will even help you lose weight.

Myth #2: "Eating cholesterol raises your cholesterol."

We have been warned that consuming too much cholesterol-rich food leads to heart disease and a plethora of other problems. This myth has resulted in foods such as whole eggs, shellfish, and saturated fats like coconut oil and animal fats being tossed aside, when actually it is inflammation that raises cholesterol.

When these highly advantageous foods are taken out of our diets, we don't get to reap the health benefits they provide. Cholesterol is a compound that is vital in helping our bodies produce hormones such as estrogen, testosterone, and cortisone. It helps build our cell membranes and the bile acids that help to digest fat. It also plays an important role in our neurological functions, including helping us form memories.

Countless studies have shown that dietary cholesterol does not significantly affect blood cholesterol levels or raise the risk of heart disease and heart attacks. We need cholesterol — our bodies actually make cholesterol, with a whopping 75% being made by our livers. Very little cholesterol found in our bodies comes from eggs, meat, or shellfish. In fact, even if we never ate any of these foods, we could still have high cholesterol simply because of our genetics. There's no reason to avoid these nutritious whole foods just because they are naturally high in cholesterol.

Lowering one's cholesterol too much can be even more dangerous than having high cholesterol. So, stop throwing out those egg yolks! If you and/ or members of your family have a history of high cholesterol, and you are concerned, you need to do more research and find a Functional Medicine doctor. Functional Medicine addresses the underlying causes of disease while considering the whole person rather than focusing on the management of isolated symptoms. Check it out.

Myth #3: "We need fiber from whole grains."

In recent years, whole grains have gone mainstream. It is not uncommon for people to opt for whole grains, because they are thought to be healthier — providing us with necessary nutrients and fiber. Wrong.

Regardless of what we've been told, most grain products actually contain very little dietary fiber. The processing of whole grains may enhance the taste and allow for a longer shelf life, but it actually strips them of antioxidants, nutrients, and — you guessed it — fiber.

On the Clean Food Diet, you get fiber from whole fruits and veggies. Even those particular whole grain foods that are thought of as rich in fiber hold no comparison to the percentages found in fruits and vegetables. A medium artichoke can contain over 10 grams of fiber at only 60 calories. Whereas a cup of brown rice has a measly 3.6 grams and almost twice the calories at 118. A cup of raspberries has about 8 grams of fiber at 64 calories, while those 2 slices of whole grain bread you're used to making a sandwich with are about 140 calories and less than 4 grams of fiber.

The fiber that comes with whole grains also comes with high calories and carb count, nasty additives, and a lot of sugar. The bottom line is that whole grains don't translate to healthy, and they certainly aren't the best source of fiber out there. So next time you're thinking about reaching for that whole grain bagel, opt for a piece of fruit or a big pile of veggies instead.

Myth #4: "We need calcium from dairy."

From health classes to advertisements, it's been drilled into our heads that we need milk in order to get enough calcium to have strong bones and teeth. Calcium, without a doubt, plays an important role in our health. However, it's a longstanding myth that we should be getting it from dairy. Dairy can actually diminish your body's calcium.

It's ironic that the words 'milk' and 'calcium' are used so interchangeably, since the calcium contained in cow's milk is barely absorbable by our bodies. While cow's milk is great for baby cows, it isn't designed for humans. And as far as strong bones go, studies have found that milk actually depletes calcium in our bones and increases the risk of fractures and osteoporosis — yikes!

It is pasteurization that kills most of the beneficial enzymes, which makes dairy tremendously difficult to digest. Thankfully, there are tons of healthy, dairy-free foods packed with calcium that can be found in the Clean Food Diet, such as collard greens, kale, turnip greens, chia seeds, fennel, broccoli, artichokes, blackberries, oranges, figs, eggs, seaweed, raspberries, and shrimp. These are just a small part of the long list of calcium-rich foods you can eat.

Myth #5: "It's better to eat six small meals a day."

In recent years, we've been told that it's healthier to eat six small meals throughout the day, rather than sticking to a breakfast, lunch, and dinner regime. The thought process behind this is that if you're continually eating smaller portions, you'll speed up your metabolism and not be as hungry or overeat. Now this whole idea of six small meals a day was actually made popular by bodybuilders who lift heavy weights for hours a day and want to acquire muscle mass. While this makes sense for them, this isn't necessarily best for everyone else.

Our bodies were meant to endure long periods of time without food. Three meals a day gives us sufficient time to burn stored body fat when needed between meals. When we continuously graze throughout the day, our bodies burn fuel from those meals, rather than from fat stores. And when that pesky fat doesn't get burned, it not only prevents us from using it as energy, but it also makes weight management much more difficult. Another benefit to sticking with three meals a day is that you're giving your body time to digest between each one.

If you're following the Clean Food Diet and eating a balance of healthy fats, carbs, and proteins during your meals, these should keep you feeling satisfied until your next meal rolls around. While three meals a day is a good rule of thumb, if you get hungry in between, that's totally ok! Don't hesitate to eat a healthy, clean snack or another clean meal.

Myth #6: "Counting calories is effective for weight loss."

We've been taught that calories-in versus calories-out is the golden rule. If you're burning more calories than you consume, then you'll lose weight, right? Well, it's not necessarily true. First of all, it's nearly impossible to accurately count calories. It's an educated guesstimate at best. Secondly, not all calories are created equal. It would be nice if losing weight and staying fit were as easy as number crunching, but unfortunately counting calories is pointless. Eating quality calories is what is effective for health and for weight loss.

If the calories you put in are junk, the output is going to be junk. Your metabolic rate along with your overall health is going to be negatively affected. For example, a cup of avocado clocks in at about 234 calories, while a chocolate bar contains 210. Sure, the chocolate is lower in calories, but it also contains 21 grams of sugar, along with preservatives and other unpronounceable additives. Not only are avocados packed with antioxidants, fiber, and protein, the monounsaturated fats within them help keep us feeling full longer and prevent us from overeating. The candy bar robs us of much needed nutrients like calcium, because our body is using them to digest the sugar. This can lead to nutritional deficiencies, weight gain, and a plethora of other health problems. Plus, it leaves us craving even more sugar, so we end up eating more and more.

You will be much better off ditching the calculator and focusing on eating whole, nutritious foods that nourish your body. Regardless of the calorie amount, when you're filling up on the whole foods found in the Clean Food Diet, you will be able to manage your weight and your body will thank you.

Myth #7: "Vegetarianism is the healthiest diet."

Well, whether it be vegetarian or vegan, going veggie has become extremely popular these days. Many people consider it to be the healthiest diet for our bodies, as well as morally superior and better for the planet. But what if I challenge that idea and am bold enough to say that according to the research that I've done, the opposite is true?

Vegetarianism, at best, lacks complete nutrition for the human body. It also may not be the best moral decision or the best idea for the planet. Now, I don't want to get into an argument with my vegetarian friends, because I used to be vegetarian for many years, and I understand that point of view. I also understand that I'm not here to change anybody. However, if you are on the fence and want to know what the optimum diet is, do the homework.

Eating a diet that is strictly plant-based is not optimum, for more reasons than we have time to go into. When we cut out meat, it's a lot harder to get enough of the essential nutrients and vitamins, like B12, Iron, and Omega-3 fatty acids, that our bodies need. And these deficiencies can cause a whole lot of problems. For starters, some of the side effects that come with going veggie are low metabolism, low body temperature, low libido, joint pain, hair loss, lack of concentration, fatigue, lack of energy, digestive issues, and bone thinning.

One of the most common reasons why people go veggie is the notion that eating meat is immoral, or that farming is bad for the environment. Well, there are a lot of humane, cruelty-free farms out there, with livestock that has been properly raised and managed, with actual benefits to the environment. But then again, please don't take my word for it.

Investigate for yourself and start the conversation.

The bottom line is that eating is a very personal act, and for some, the decision is based on cultural and religious traditions. Let's just all agree to let each person decide for themselves what makes them feel, look, and perform better.

If you are ready to take on the Clean Food Challenge for 21 days and see how it works for you, go to www.MasterMel.com/CFD for more resources and support. Let me help you get started today!

About Melodee Meyer

Melodee Meyer, aka Master Mel, is an international bestselling author, speaker, radio host, and mentor, who has taught thousands of folks how to love themselves lean, fit, and healthy. Her Self Mastery System empowers hungry leaders and passionate entrepreneurs to create the life they want, in a body they love, so they can go out and change the world.

Overcoming challenges in her own life, including bullying, bulimia, domestic abuse, and life as a single mom, Master Mel uses her expertise in martial arts, psychology, health, and fitness to work with women and organizations who are ready for the next level of mastery in their lives. (Is that you?)

Melodee received her Master's Degree in Spiritual Psychology; is a Certified Nutritional Consultant; and is a 5th Dan Black Belt, recently inducted into the Karate Union Hall of Fame. She developed the award-winning fitness program, Kickboxers Ultimate Training (getKUT.com); is the creator of Clean KUT Nutrition (Whey Clean Protein supplement available at CleanKUT.com); and the founder of Self Mastery Bootcamp.

Melodee loves to cook, eat, and take pictures of food. (Yes, it's an obsession.) She also loves to livestream, write, teach, and play at Martial Arts Family Fitness, a center she owns with her family in Santa Barbara, California.

To book Melodee Meyer to speak at your next event, or to get more information about the Clean Food Diet, feeding yourself PIES or the Self Mastery System, visit MasterMel.com.

Book MASTER MEL to Speak

You're Guaranteed to Make Your Next Event Unforgettable With Keynote Speaker Melodee Meyer

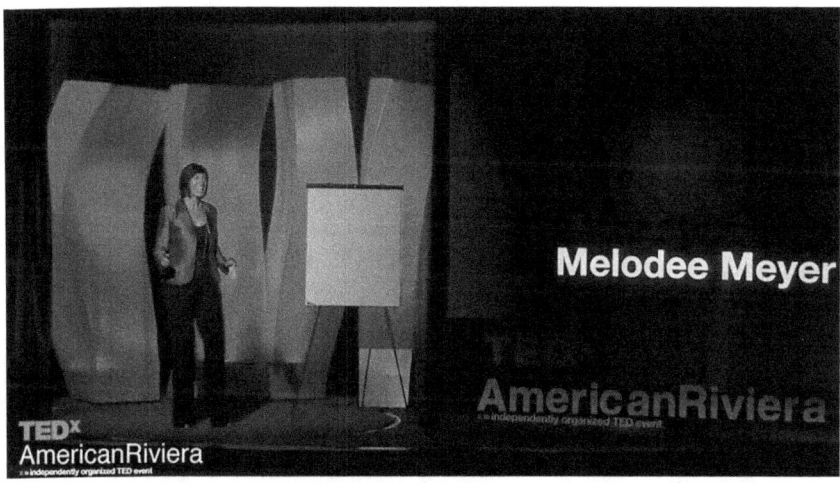

For years, Melodee Meyer has been educating, entertaining and inspiring entrepreneurs, leaders, women's groups, executives and business owners to confidently step into their power so they can live the life they want, in a body they love, doing work that matters.

Melodee's personal journey from abuse victim to martial arts master will leave your audience with specific and practical tools that will empower them to take action on their dreams and achieve their next level of success NOW, at work or at home.

For more information and to book Melodee for your next event,
visit **www.MasterMel.com/speaker**

or call/text

(805) 699-6757